EMOTIONAL INTELLIGENCE MASTERY: DEVELOP SELF DISCIPLINE, OVERCOME PROCRASTINATION & OVERTHINKING (4 IN 1)

MASTER YOUR EMOTIONS, BUILD POSITIVE HABITS & MENTAL TOUGHNESS TO REACH YOUR FULL POTENTIAL

STEWART HUNTER

DEVON HOUSE
PRESS

CONTENTS

SELF-DISCIPLINE & MENTAL TOUGHNESS FOR SUCCESS & HAPPINESS (2 IN 1)

OVERCOME PROCRASTINATION & OVERTHINKING (2 IN 1)

SELF-DISCIPLINE & MENTAL TOUGHNESS FOR SUCCESS & HAPPINESS (2 IN 1)

DEVELOP YOUR DISCIPLINE, BUILD HEALTHY
DAILY HABITS & OVERCOME
PROCRASTINATION TO FULFIL YOUR
POTENTIAL & FIND TRUE FREEDOM

I

THE ROAD TO SELF-DISCIPLINE AND MENTAL TOUGHNESS

A FULL DIVE ON WHAT YOU'RE AIMING FOR

We begin the journey towards better self-discipline and mental toughness by taking a look at what we're looking to do. In this chapter, we're going to dive into what discipline is, and how you should view it.

We'll also discuss whether or not mental toughness is something to rely on for everyday things or in times where the pressure is on and you won't settle for anything less than your best. We'll discuss more about the definition of mental toughness and how its viewed (while comparing it to how it should be viewed).

Every journey is not easy. And you will come across some obstacles as you travel from Point A to Point B. No one is born with discipline and mental toughness.

This book will show you how to build on those things from the ground up. Now, let's talk a bit about discipline.

WHAT DOES IT MEAN TO BE DISCIPLINED?

Discipline is something that is taught. It's not something that we're born with. Discipline means being able to perform a task whether you like to do it or not. If you set up some rules and standards that you want to adhere by, following them will be defined as discipline.

For example, let's say you want to be out of bed by 5AM. You learn to discipline yourself by getting up at that time even if the idea of sleeping in another hour is tempting. Being disciplined means you're behaving in a certain way.

But why is it that people view discipline as some "bad word"? We'll explain that in the next section.

DISCIPLINE SOUNDS LIKE...SO HOW IS IT DIFFERENT?

Most people view discipline as a bad thing. Specifically, the word "discipline" is anchored to the event when someone does something wrong (like stealing cookies from the cookie jar), they need to be disciplined for it. However, the use of the word is in a different context.

You won't be grounded for a month for being lazy or having a poor mindset. The kind of discipline we are aiming for is in the context of restraining yourself. If there is something you need to scale back on or quit entirely (bad habits and such), you'll need to discipline yourself.

You need to restrain yourself from something that may hold power over you. Allowing yourself to give into vices will not only validate the fact that you are giving power to it, but it proves that your level of discipline or restraint is low.

Not giving in is a sure sign of strength. Especially when we're talking about mental strength and toughness. But why is it so hard to do?

The rewards of being disciplined and restraining yourself from making bad decisions is within easy reach. It's like a pot of gold sitting in front of you just waiting to be claimed by you. Yet, somehow, we make it impossible to achieve it.

We tend to get comfortable with our bad habits and vices. And depending on what it is, we pay the price for it thanks to short-term and long-term effects. For example, let's take a look at procrastination.

You have a big project coming up. The deadline is a few weeks out. The sooner you get it done, the better.

But you decide to put it off because you have a comfortable amount of time to "goof off" before the due date. So, you say to yourself "Screw it. It can wait". You do some of your favorite things like play video games, veg out on the couch and watch Netflix, or whatever else.

Before you know it, two weeks pass and suddenly you're under a lot of pressure to finish the project. You allow the pressure to get to you mentally and you feel like you're about to go crazy. You sacrifice sleep, put off other important things, and what have you.

You soon come to the realization that had you got this done sooner, perhaps you wouldn't feel like a zombie for a few days. You put things off that you think you're going to do tomorrow (but never do until the last minute). Now let's compare that to the other way around.

Close your eyes for a moment. Imagine you have already read this book, adopted the principles you've learned to become more disciplined and mentally tough. Now, let's replay that same scenario.

You have a project coming up. It's due a few weeks from now. You think to yourself, perfect maybe I can get it out of the way so I can do what I want in my free time. So, you chip away at the project on day one.

You pace yourself and take your time. You're not in a rush to get it done (and if you did that, the quality would show for it). You spend a few hours per day while ignoring texts, Facebook notifications, and so on.

One of the notifications on your phone unbeknownst to you is some update of your favorite game. You probably don't care at this point because you have more important things to do. Sometimes, procrastinating can work in your favor when it's something that tends to be a distraction (but we digress).

So, a week and a half has passed. The project is done and ahead of schedule. Sure, you decided to stay up a little later because you had so much fun doing something that keeps you busy.

The quality is impressive. Nothing is half-assed. And your boss, client, project partners, or colleagues are quite happy with the amount of effort and detail you put into it.

The work shows that you cared about investing your time wisely in the important things. That gives you a level of unmatchable confidence. And it boosts your mental toughness in the process.

That's because you've learned how to discipline yourself by placing priorities over all else. You've put the interests of others over yourself (not in a pushover sort of way). Someone wanted to get a project done and you managed to put in the time and effort to help them out.

As a result, you are handsomely rewarded for all of your efforts (and get a nice pay bonus as the cherry on top). Will discipline and mental toughness earn you a raise at your job? We can't guarantee that.

But we can say that discipline and mental toughness does have its rewards. When you are able to restrain yourself from making poor decisions, you will feel good about it mentally. Your level of discipline will not only affect you, but it will affect others as well.

For example, if the project you did is in poor quality then it will affect the people you work with. The client will view your company unfavorably and may shift gears and work with someone else. This will tarnish your company's image and it can lead to some tough decisions for your boss both in the short-term and long-term (which may include cutting you loose as part of the cutback process so their company stays afloat).

Discipline, whether you have it or lack it, will trigger a domino effect like nothing else. That is why discipline is so important. If you fail to use it, who knows what kind of effect it will have on you and others in a negative way.

HOW RELIABLE IS MENTAL TOUGHNESS?

Mental toughness is usually a term that we hear in sports. One of the biggest proponents of it is Bill Belichick. And it's one of the core reasons why the New England Patriots had been one of the most successful teams in football history winning a total of six Super Bowl titles.

Belichick said the following: "Mental toughness is continuing to do the right things even when things aren't going right for you personally". Read that last sentence again. Hammer meets nail.

The truth is, discipline and mental toughness go hand in hand. There are some things that have to get done, but you're having a bad day and you'd rather just lay on the couch, relax, and forget about everything. You could be having the worst day ever, but it's incumbent upon you to do your part even if you don't feel like it.

Let's take a look at another example where mental toughness and discipline go together. Suppose you are just reading through a comment thread on social media. And someone decided to get nasty with someone based on some difference in opinion.

You read the comment and the temptation to fire back an angry and equally nasty reply appears. Mind you, the comment wasn't directly towards you. You have the choice to just ignore it and move on (even if it goes against what you feel you should do personally) or get sucked right in and prove yourself that like the dimwit who left the nasty comment, you are as undisciplined and not as mentally tough.

The truth is anyone who tries to engage in these comment wars by putting down someone is lacking in discipline and mental toughness. What bothered them to get to that point? It's true what they say: don't stoop down to their level (in this case, their level of mental toughness and discipline...which is lacking).

Is mental toughness reliable? The answer is yes. It's only unreliable if you choose not to use it.

Mental toughness is built so you can consistently perform at a level where you can get the job done and never compromise on quality. Mental toughness allows you to fine tune yourself and get better. And it protects your level of success now and in the future.

You don't have to always rely on talent. You rely on your consistency, your willingness to work hard, and let nothing get in the way of your goals (whether they are short-term or long-term goals). Mental toughness is an element that is needed in leadership.

Like discipline, mental toughness will affect others in a positive way. Specifically, mentally tough leaders will have the backs of those who follow them. They will build them up and encourage them to do better (as opposed to talk them down).

When a leader gets the team going, they work together as one mentally tough unit and achieve that one common goal they want.

Case in point, Bill Belichick's leadership (and his "Patriot Way" of discipline) led to the number of Super Bowl titles and cementing himself into one of football's greatest coaches.

MENTAL TOUGHNESS SOUNDS LIKE…SO HOW IS IT DIFFERENT?

When people think of mental toughness, they think it sounds like this: Be tough, show no emotion, and keep doing what you do. In other words, don't let anyone see you cry or get angry. Just get on with it like some emotionless robot.

Thais couldn't be farther from the truth. You shouldn't withhold emotions. If you are going through a rough day, it's okay to use that emotion to get through the pain.

It's okay to cry when you've had a rough day. And it doesn't matter if anyone sees it or not. And it's okay to voice your frustrations and anger.

As long as you keep yourself in check and never let it get out of control, invoking negative emotions to get through the pain will help you become mentally tougher. You can make a more positive impression if you know how to maintain a positive attitude while managing your emotions at a healthy level (compared to being an emotionless robot, which makes you look bland and boring).

What mental toughness should actually sound like is having a positive mindset. You're accepting of the fact that failure will happen multiple times. When it does, you should move forward with a sense of knowing that things will go well in the future.

Failure is not an indication that it's the end of the world. Nor is it an indicator that you should give up and resign to a life of mediocrity or whatever else. Also, managing your own stress in stressful situations is also a defining pillar in mental toughness.

Regardless if things are going wrong or when the pressure is on, the last thing you want to do is fold and give up. Even when working through the stress, there will always be a reward at the end of the tunnel. And that sense of accomplishment will give you the dopamine rush you deserve.

Mental toughness is built on the following four pillars: Challenge, Control, Commitment, and Confidence. When things get challenging, you'll want to be in control with as much of it as possible. See it through to the end and you'll have the confidence in conquering every single challenge you face.

Control is the most important of the four. Either you control the stress and pressure, or it controls you. You have the power to rise above any challenge, so don't let it be the other way around.

LIKE EVERY OTHER ROAD IN OUR LIFE, IT'S BOUND TO GET BUMPY

It's true what they say: there are roads in life that will get bumpy. Some of them will have obstacles that will be challenging to navigate. But that's all part of the journey.

It's a road less traveled. But unbeknownst to most is that you get to your destination faster. Before you say anything else, this road is no shortcut.

Compare that to another road. It's smooth, flat, and has plenty of light. You see it as far as the horizon.

Does it go to the same destination? Yes, it does. Nothing in the way, no roadblocks, no obstacles.

Seems simple enough to travel on it, right? What could possibly go wrong? You travel down the road and get to the end when suddenly you find yourself falling a thousand feet below.

It's irrefutable proof that what can go wrong, will go wrong. Things can go "smoothly" and suddenly you drop off and lose control. You survive the fall miraculously. But the journey gets a lot tougher (not to mention it takes a longer period of time to get to your destination).

Simply put, you can choose to accept the fact that there will be challenges and bumpy roads along the way. Or you can take the "easy" route and suddenly see yourself falling off a "Cliff" when you least expect it.

Now that you are aware of this, the question you'll be asking yourself on a regular basis is "where do I go from here"? If you see yourself stuck on this bumpy road and you have a hard time navigating the obstacles, you can always ask for help.

It's easy for us to be stubborn and eschew the idea for fear of embarrassment. But no one has ever died from asking someone for help on how to get from one point to the next in their journey towards self-discipline and mental toughness. Seek out the people who you believe are the most disciplined and mentally toughest people you know and ask questions.

At that point, you can learn from them about their own journey that helped them build their self-discipline and mental toughness. They've been there and done that. They know the roads are full of bumps and potholes.

Do you have to copy everything down to the letter of what they need? Not really. But you can find some excellent nuggets of advice and ideas to help you better navigate the obstacles while traveling the rough roads towards self-discipline and mental toughness.

RECAP

At this point, you already know the real truth about discipline and mental toughness. We've already debunked the age-old myths that discipline is a bad thing. And that mental toughness doesn't mean being an emotionless robot either.

Discipline is where restraint comes into play when something that holds enough power to suck you in to do the opposite of what you want. It's easy for us to get that extra half hour of sleep. Or to rest on our laurels for hours on end and binge watch our favorite shows on Netflix.

Your lack of discipline is something that not only will affect you, but it will affect other people as well. It's a domino effect like nothing else.

Discipline and mental toughness indeed go hand in hand (especially when control is one of the key blocks to the latter).

In order to establish discipline and mental toughness, it's all about having control. Either you control yourself or let the vices of procrastination and bad habits control you. On top of that, you'll need to be aware that challenges will exist.

It will be up to you to conquer those challenges while managing your stress at the same time. You'll see it through to the end no matter how many obstacles you face. When you conquer the challenges, you increase your confidence.

The more confidence you have, beating the challenges will be as easy and effortless as ordering your favorite pizza. Now that you have a full dive on what we're aiming for, it's time to identify the obstacles that stand in the way.

In the next chapter, we'll be covering several common roadblocks and obstacles that you may have encountered (and will likely do so again) when you're on the journey towards discipline and mental toughness. Strap in, turn the page, and let's go for a ride.

II

WHAT'S GETTING IN YOUR WAY

YOUR #1 ENEMY IS YOURSELF

Pow! Right away, we kick off this chapter with a knock into reality. Like the name of the chapter, the number one enemy, your archnemesis in achieving self-discipline and mental toughness is none other than yourself. There really is no point in blaming anyone else or situation for this.

It's easy to blame someone for things. Especially when it comes to a lack of discipline and mental weakness. In fact, it's a major symptom of both.

In this chapter, we're going to talk about what makes you public enemy number one when it comes to this ultimate goal we are trying to achieve. We've also got one more little surprise to spring on you (and to warn you, it's kind of an unwelcome one). Once you find out what it is, we'll discuss what you can do about it so you can be on the path to positive instead of walking around in negative circles.

Now that you know that you are your own worst enemy in terms of trying to be more disciplined and mentally tough, let's get to the common issues that make that happen (even if you don't know about them already):

YOUR PRIORITIES ARE ALL OVER THE PLACE AND YOU CAN'T FOCUS ON ONE THING

Of course, this is common for almost everyone. We tend to work on one thing then shift to the next thing ten seconds later and repeat the process. It's a vicious never-ending cycle.

It's easy for us to lose attention with one task because we're now paying attention to one other thing. But that amount of attention that task is getting is short-lived and fleeting because we see yet another thing to pay attention to. Before we know it, we lose track of it all and it's nothing more than a huge confusing mess.

The key word here is prioritization. It's about putting the most critical task first among others before the other. So why is it so hard to do?

That's because we mix our priorities with our personal goals. Sure, those goals are important. But there are things that have to be done beforehand.

You'll want to plan out your clear priorities before the day begins. And there are a few reasons why that is:

- With clear, planned out priorities you can be able to structure your day. You get the most critical task done before moving onto the next one. Some things have to be done and the window is tight in terms of deadlines. The closer the deadline, the more critical it is.

- It will show you how to effectively use the words "yes" and "no". Regarding the latter, you're going to learn how to say it without breaking a sweat or stressing about it. You'll need to learn how to say "no" to things that are not as urgent nor important. We'll explain this further in the chapter.

- You'll be investing your time wisely and sort of by force (depending on how critical the task is). With a set plan with your priorities ahead of the pack, you'll know exactly where to spend your time and how long. Not to mention, you will be prepared to get the task done without sacrificing any quality. Keep in mind that there is little to no room for half-assing it.

- You'll learn how to focus on ONE task at a time. Sure, people will say that they are good at multitasking. Just because they say it doesn't mean you have to do it either. In fact, resist the urge to attempt multi-tasking as much as possible. You're only human and you can only do as much as possible. Instead of multitasking, delegate if necessary.

One of the best ways to plan and prioritize your tasks is to take a page out of Dwight D. Eisenhower, a military leader who later became President of the United States. Eisenhower devised a way to put his most critical tasks ahead of everything else.

This became known as the Eisenhower Matrix. To get a sense of what this looks like, pay attention to the following chart:

Urgent/Important	Do or don't do?
Urgent AND Important	Do
Urgent BUT Not Important	Delegate (but do if time allows it)
Not urgent BUT Important	Do it, but at a later time
Not urgent AND Not Important	Don't do it

The Eisenhower Matrix is separated into four quadrants determined on urgency and importance. If the task is urgent and important, that is your most critical task. And it must be done before all else.

If the task is urgent but not important, you will likely opt to delegate to someone who can get it done for you (assuming the level of urgency is high). If you are lucky enough to have a small enough time window to get it done, go for it. But use your better judgement in such a situation.

Next is not urgent but important. Indeed, these tasks are important enough for you to pay attention to. However, the timing of getting them down is not as urgent. You could schedule to get it done the following day or the day after.

Lastly, we have the not urgent and not important things. This is where a lot of people are. They do the tasks that cause us to procrastinate and blow off other tasks that hold a lot more priority.

In this instance, you'll want to be disciplined enough to know that saying no to these tasks is fine. It won't be the be all to end all. Also, you'll want to learn the words "not now" in terms of those not urgent but important tasks.

The truth is you need to pay close attention to your most critical tasks (your urgent AND important tasks). The last thing you want to ever do is pull a slight amount of attention and time away from it. Do it once and you'll be sucked into the vortex of doing something else that holds little to no priority over the task at hand.

Use the Eisenhower Matrix to place your most critical tasks in the URGENT and IMPORTANT quadrant first while planning out the day. Then schedule the URGENT and NOT IMPORTANT next, followed by NOT URGENT but IMPORTANT last.

THE TENDENCY TO OVERTHINK AND IMAGINE THE WORSE

Ah yes. Overthinking. If that isn't one of the most serious symptoms of doing nothing, we don't know what is. But what exactly causes overthinking?

Believe it or not, there are a few things that overthinking can stem from. Let's cut to the chase and identify them:

- **Past mistakes:** People make mistakes. That's just the undeniable truth. But the real problem is because of them, most people are afraid to do something again. They fear that they'll mess up on something and it will turn out less than perfect. They fear failure (and deem it as an opportunity to give up and move one).

- **You play the same scene in your head repeatedly:**
  Suppose you have a presentation coming up. This is the big
  one where you land a big client if you succeed. And if you
  make one mistake, it will cost you. The "what ifs of things
  gone wrong" tend to pop up. It's okay to practice and
  rehearse the presentation to iron out the wrinkles. In fact,
  overthinking will suck up plenty of time that should
  otherwise go towards rehearsing your presentation. And if
  you make a mistake, don't make a big deal out of it. Act as if
  it never happened and move on.

- **You focus on the "worst case scenario":** Visualization
  is a great preparedness tool. And there is nothing wrong
  with it. However, visualizing the worst that could happen
  will mentally overpower you to a point where fear of failure
  will settle in. Instead of focusing on the worst, focus on the
  best-case scenario. The more you visualize it and practice it,
  the better off you'll be. Also, don't worry about perfection.
  Just rehearse as if you are going through the motions.

- **Worrying about things beyond your control:**
  Everybody worries about things. Especially when it's things
  they can't change nor control. It's not your fault that a nasty
  thunderstorm knocked out power and left the city in the
  dark. Nor is it your fault if some dastardly cyber villain hacks
  into the computer network at the office, which also
  complicates things in the process. Another thing beyond
  your control is someone else's decision making. You can
  persuade someone to make a decision to an extent. However,
  if they don't follow through then don't worry about it. It's

their decision and you can't blame them for it. On the bright side, it could be the worst decision they've made, and they'll come to regret it sooner rather than later.

WHY OVERTHINKING IS BAD

If you think overthinking is some kind of minor thing, you'd actually be surprised. Overthinking may place a negative role in your mental psyche. In fact, it could trigger mental illnesses that may cause you to lose your sanity and peace of mind.

Not only that, but overthinking will make problem solving even harder. It can even make solving the most basic problem that can be solved in five seconds even more complex. It's hard to imagine that ever happening to someone.

Last but certainly not least, it can also affect your sleep patterns. It's good to have a sharp and clear mind when you are well rested. But overthinking will be the biggest obstacle in making that happen.

It will turn what could otherwise be 7 to 9 hours of sleep into 3 to 4 hours. And that's the last thing you want to deal with any day of the week.

How to "kill" your overthinking

So, how do you go about dispatching your overthinking with extreme prejudice? What you may not know is that there are simple solutions. Here are some things we highly recommend you do to ensure that overthinking is a thing of the past:

Know what you can control and what you can't: Accepting the fact that you can't change or control the things that are beyond you is what you need to do. Things that are not directly associated with you will always happen. It's always good to be prepared to be slightly ahead of the curve when things go south.

For example, if you are doing a PowerPoint presentation, have some hard copies handy in the event of the computer you use mysteriously dying. Just shrug it off as another one of those things that you can't control, hand the people you're presenting the hard copies and lead them in a follow along. Not only will they be impressed with how you handled such a situation, but they will love that someone took the initiative to stay ahead of Murphy's Law.

Optimism is key: If you fail, it won't be the end of the world. Think to yourself that one day, there will be a favorable outcome. That one day could come tomorrow, six months from now, or next year. It will happen. Don't let failure be the end all to be all.

Cheer for yourself: It's easy for us to be hard on ourselves. But that will really embed some negative seeds in your mindset. Instead, you can be your own best cheerleader. Even if no one believes in what you can do, you are your best believer. And that alone sets you a head above shoulders over those who don't think this way.

Learn to meditate: There is nothing more satisfying than meditation. No, you don't have to close your eyes and chant "omm" every minute. You can do it quietly in a separate space where no one can bother you. We also would be remiss if we didn't suggest any guided meditation apps like Calm or Headspace. Also, some guided meditation videos on YouTube will always come in handy. You could also incorporate it in your daily routine. It doesn't have to be long. Just block off five minutes of your day and try it out.

With your ability to eliminate overthinking with little to no effort, you have one of the key skills that will no doubt set you apart from those who lack discipline and mental toughness. Restraining yourself from negative thoughts and self-doubt is a powerful skill that will show through your body language and the way you behave.

There is no tricking your subconscious. If you have a positive inner mindset and you train your brain not to overthink, people will know a mentally strong and self-disciplined individual without even asking a single question.

JUST ADMIT IT, YOU DON'T LIKE RESPONSIBILITY

We're not trying to sound rude or anything. A lot of us are not huge fans of responsibility. And you are more than likely one of them.

Just know that you are not alone in this sentiment. People hate being able to own up to things. And that's where it's easy to blame others even though you know deep down that you're at fault.

People seem to avoid responsibility like the plague. Responsibility itself is like a bloodhound. It doesn't matter how much you shake it off, it will hunt you down and find out where you're hiding soon enough. So, you might as well take on responsibilities when the opportunity presents itself.

Learning how to take responsibility for things must be taught at an early enough age. Being responsible will help strengthen your wellbeing, your decision making, and how productive you can be. On top of that, responsibility will also help you strengthen yourself in times when you'll be making certain decisions.

Specifically, these are decisions that won't go over well with others. But they are the kind of decisions that will be for a greater good. For example, you're an executive who is faced with the responsibility of laying off one of two people due to cutbacks.

You know that making such a decision can save the company money. However, your decision may decide the fate of someone who has been a loyal and dedicated employee for a number of years. It will alter the course of their life for the long term.

You need to swallow hard, make a choice, and move forward.

Why no one wants to be held liable

Being held liable may sound like a legal term. Yet, in this context we are discussing liability in terms of what happens when the outcome is negative. There isn't a single person alive who would want a negative outcome.

They happen all the time. But the real issue lies in how one person will handle it. Will they handle the negative outcome with optimism and treat it like a learning lesson? Or will they lay blame on something or someone knowing full well the outcome may have been well in their control?

There are a few reasons why people do the latter: one, they are afraid of failure. Or in plain English, they don't know how to handle it properly. Second, they are not confident in their abilities. And lastly, they choose not to be involved in as much of the process as possible.

So, they decide to hang back behind the scenes and do nothing for fear that if things go wrong, it's their fault. Inaction will earn you a share of the blame, so avoiding liability won't help you.

The fear of failure or lack of confidence will serve as an excuse. The doing of a task will be enough to help you gain the confidence in going forward next time, whether you fail or not. And once again, failure is not the be all to end all.

If you give it your best and it results in the negative, it's important to take a look at what went wrong, discuss what could have been done differently, and move on. Also, people will blame you for the failure (which you shouldn't take personally). People who blame others is a sign of the inability to handle failure on their own accord.

The inability to handle failure and place blame on others will affect the overall morale and mentality of others. That will make it hard for a group to work together on future projects or the like. Learn how to handle failure together if such a thing occurs.

The "diffusion of responsibility"

In a team setting, there may be someone who might be blindly following orders or instructions without knowing what it all entails. That person will usually stand idle and wait for someone to make a move. This is known as the "diffusion of responsibility".

The person who does this needs to take action without waiting for someone else to make the move. Not only that, but it places the other team members in a pressure situation where someone has to make the move. Don't let any lack of initiative come down to that.

The "Yes" Syndrome

It's always a good idea to know your limits. You'll want to learn how to say "yes" to the right responsibilities. On top of that, you'll need to learn how to take on things one at a time rather than overload yourself.

Overloading yourself with responsibilities will overwhelm you. And you may freeze up as a result. You'll begin to panic, overthink, and worry more about what needs to get done first.

This alone will throw everything into chaos. You will soon lose track of what needs to get done. And it will mentally burn you out.

Do not do this to yourself. Know what you are capable of and perform your responsibilities accordingly. Don't feel pressured to say "yes" to all of them.

Learn to say "no", explain your reason why (and make it a good one), and move on.

UNBEKNOWNST TO YOU, YOU'VE ALREADY DEVELOPED FALSE HOPE SYNDROME

Remember that surprise we mentioned earlier on in the chapter? Well, here it is. Whether you know it or not (and it's likely the latter), you already developed what is known as false hope syndrome.

To give you a prime example of this in action, let's talk about New Year's Resolutions. Every year, we vow to make a change for a greater good. It can be losing weight, making more money, quitting smoking, or whatever else.

The real problem is that we fail to fulfill this resolution. Why is this exactly? There is no specific goal that is set. Not to mention, it's lacking in structure.

It's easy for us to adopt the old "go big or go home" mentality. Yet, a lot of us don't seem to know how to set small, tangible goals to get to a much larger one. So instead of "losing weight", just say you're planning on losing 20 pounds.

Then you can outline how to get there. You'll have small milestone goals that you can attain throughout the year. And there is also one thing to keep in mind, set the goals you want to achieve based on your own values.

You're probably scratching your head at that last part. Let's explain it in better detail. Let's say for instance, you want to quit drinking soda or coffee. But there is one thing that stands in your way.

You place a high value on caffeine, which helps you stay awake and alert. Getting rid of coffee or soda will cause you to cut off one of the things you value most. And depriving yourself of things that are personally valuable to you will lead to eventual failure (and giving up your resolutions even before the old groundhog pops up and checks for his shadow).

When settling your goals, consider how it will affect your personal values. If caffeine is really that important, you'll want to explore alternatives that will ensure you still get the caffeine you need without having to resort to anything unhealthy.

If you drink a copious amount of soda on a regular basis, consider cutting that out of your diet. Instead, drink coffee or caffeinated tea. If it's difficult to give up on soda, consider diet or sugar free options. Making changes without hurting your values is possible.

Figure out what is standing in the way

If you are looking for a way to reach a goal or resolution, it's all about identifying the obstacles that stand in the way. Let's say you had a new year's resolution and you failed to fulfill it. What happened? What stood in the way?

Furthermore, ask yourself what you could have done differently. For example, let's circle back to the weight loss goal. You want to spend time working out, so you decide to at least try and do it in the morning before work.

However, you find that your window of time isn't enough, so you give up on it and blame it on a lack of time. Instead of doing that, you should consider blocking off a specific period of time. Why not work out after the workday? It can be as simple as going home, lifting and swinging a kettlebell for 15 to 20 minutes and calling it a day.

Know your values and stay true to them

Your values can either work together or work against each other. That's another reason why people find giving up their goals and resolutions easily. It's important to know what they are and stay true to them as much as possible.

You'll also want to try and mitigate any potential clashes as much as possible. Losing weight while eating to handle stress is counteractive to your goals. So, find an alternative to handle and alleviate stress. Believe it or not, working out is a great stress blaster if we say so ourselves.

Plus, you can use that stress as an energy source to put in the work without killing yourself. You'll feel good knowing that you've utilized that stress to your advantage and decided to knock out some calories in the process. You'll be a lean mean machine that is mentally tough, disciplined, and has a fool-proof way to handle stress when the going gets rough.

Will you always be working out every time you're in a stressful situation? Not always. So, it's important to find other stress management techniques as well.

As long as it's within your own personal values and the results don't counteract with the benefits, you should be in good shape.

YOU END UP DOING SOMETHING ELSE AND YOU STILL KEEP ON JUSTIFYING YOUR ACTIONS

When we end up doing one thing or another, it's easy for us to justify our actions. We make mistakes and we try to explain why we did them. Self-justification is a little more dangerous than any of us would imagine.

We defend our actions or mistakes as if it were one of those "I had to do what was best" moments. It's easy for us to make excuses when we can't give ourselves a straight answer (or to anyone else for that matter).

If you screw up on something and it can be salvageable, the best time to start is right now. Don't wait until tomorrow, next week, or next month. If you screw up and you have an opportunity to start over, jump on it at the earliest time possible (which obviously is now).

One of the top killers for self-discipline is making excuses for yourself. The only way you can stop making excuses is to own up to your mistakes, promise yourself to do better, and say that it can be done.

Self-justifying our actions is equivalent to defending someone who committed a heinous act (even though you know they did it). How can someone you look up to as a mentor be a good person when behind closed doors, they are abusive to their spouse? How can someone be a good person in the face of the public but in private, they are plotting to exploit and scam the same people out of their hard-earned money?

There is no such thing as doing wrong and making yourself look good in the process. This is one of the sure signs of someone who is lacking in discipline and mental toughness. Try as they may, once their house of cards finally falls, they have no choice but to cower in fear and never be seen or heard from again.

Justifying procrastination

Here's the thing with procrastination: you put off something that can be done today, but you'll do it tomorrow. One of the things that is usually said to justify this behavior is "I've got plenty of time throughout the day. I'll do it later". Thus, they'd rather invest their time on other things they think are important all while that time window of doing that exact task is shrinking fast.

Sure, a project that's due two weeks from now is plenty of time. But the sooner you get it done, the better. That way, you can use that spare time to focus on other things or relax (assuming there's nothing else).

NARCISSISTS: LACKING ONE THING, BUT NOT THE OTHER

If someone continues to justify their actions and repeatedly do the same bad things without shame, then that's a sign of narcissism. Here's a plot twist that will shock you: believe it or not, while narcissistic people tend to do wrong and justify their actions, they are mentally tough themselves.

But we're not teaching you to become narcissistic. They are using this power as a weapon of mass destruction. We're showing you how to use it for a greater good.

You see, narcissists use mental toughness to shield themselves from the negativity generated from the people they knowingly hurt and harm. They justify and explain their actions as if it were the right thing (when in reality they know they're wrong). But they don't care.

They lack discipline, but they don't care either. Despite the fact they are mentally tough, they are undisciplined. They will refuse to own up to their mistakes and will place the blame on others.

Lucky for you, this book does give you the keys to being a self-disciplined and mentally tough individual. Unlike the narcissists we speak of, you'll be miles ahead of them in terms of owning your mistakes, learning from them, placing the blame on yourself, and moving forward.

This will help you cultivate a positive self-image in the eyes of your friends, family, and colleagues. You can't be mentally tough and undisciplined, nor be disciplined but not mentally tough. It can't be done.

HOW TO "KILL" SELF-JUSTIFICATION

We can make a decision without thinking twice and be faced with dire consequences. For example, you may be a manager of a small business and make decisions based on cutting back due to financial strain. However, you recklessly make such decisions here or there without the knowledge or input of the employees or customers.

Doing this and saying "it's for the benefit of the company" isn't going to win over anyone. So, how do you go about making the right decisions while killing any opportunity at self-justification? Here are some tips to consider in the long run:

Think it over and ask someone: If you are considering making a decision that carries some serious weight, it's important to not jump on it just yet. It's good to take your time, weigh the pros and cons, and find out who it could affect the most. Ask your most trusted friends, members of your family, or your closest colleagues about what you're considering doing. Ask them about the upsides and downsides. It's better to talk it out and find out what would be the best or worst scenario should it go forward.

Surround yourself with the right people: In this context, the right people are those who will have no problem disagreeing with you. When someone disagrees with you on a potential decision, they are more than likely doing you a favor. They could be saving you from making a fatal error that can never be reversed. They'll also aid you in righting the ship before things get worse. If you are in a leadership position, it's never a good idea to be surrounded by people who will say "yes" 100 percent of the time.

Keep your emotions in check: When decisions are made at high levels of emotion, the likelihood of disaster will be even greater. That's why it is important to put together a plan where you'll need to make the most difficult decisions while keeping the levels of emotion as low as possible. In situations where you're negotiating with the other side on a huge deal or when you decide who gets what in your will when you pass away, you'll want to use more logic than emotion.

Don't use self-justification language: "What about" ..." It's legal" ..." I couldn't do it because" ...these are just a sample of self-justification language. It's important you catch on what you say and use an alternative that doesn't put you in a position of justifying a bad decision.

Don't arrive at conclusions early: Before you even know the real facts, don't arrive at a conclusion. When new information arises, you'll be forced to walk back what you say. And it will make you look bad. Plus, it creates the perfect climate for self-justification.

The sooner you own your mistakes, the better: Why lie to yourself? Why lie to others? When you know you've made a mistake, admit it and move forward. Don't drag it out any farther than you have to.

Assess the situation: It's important to assess a certain situation that you find yourself in. Ask yourself what role you played. Also, ask yourself what could have been done to make it better even if someone is to blame for it (including yourself).

Simply put, a true cornerstone of self-discipline and mental toughness is knowing that it's okay to admit to your mistakes. It won't make you a failure and it certainly won't view you in a more negative manner (unlike denying it, blaming others, and moving on). Resist the urge to place the blame on others, self-justifying decisions that were never right to begin with, and acting as if nothing happened and no one got hurt.

YOU ARE NOT TAKING CARE OF YOURSELF

Whether you know it or not, your lack of discipline and mental toughness can take a toll in more ways than one. Specifically, we're talking about your overall physical health. The truth is, a lack of discipline and mental toughness may lead to some not so good decisions.

Sure, it's nice to treat ourselves with a McDonald's combo meal here and there. But eating fast food on the regular will likely do more harm than good. Especially when it's food that is high in fats, sodium, calories, and so on.

But in this context, the question we need to ask ourselves is: Are we taking care of ourselves mentally? The lack of concentration and focus can lead us down some paths that may not allow us to turn back.

If you are consistently lacking concentration and focus, it can be tied to a few factors. For one, a lack of sleep can lead to it. Aside from that, a lack of sleep can also lead to adverse effects on your physical health as well. As we have hinted earlier, a poor diet can do more harm than good.

Eating the wrong foods on a regular basis can also lead to a lack of concentration and focus as well. It would be better for you to consider making some changes in your diet. Anything high in sugar (for example) will give you that temporary energy and high before you crash back down, and you feel tired.

Also, being stressed all the time will lead to health problems as well. When you are stressed, you can forget about concentration and focus. Stress is like a needle that will keep pricking and poking you to a point where it can be very bothersome. That will throw you off course on the tasks at hand and you'll be pulled away to focus on something that's bothering you more than it should.

Believe it or not, there are medical conditions where a lack of focus and concentration can occur (such as ADHD, diabetes, or even depression). It can also be a symptom of something that could be much worse.

(Note: We are not medical professionals. And we are not in the authority to give you sound medical advice. If you lack focus or concentration and suffer other symptoms like severe chest pains, severe headaches, disorientation, or other signs of a serious condition consult a medical professional immediately. While we talk of putting things off until later, doing so in this situation can have fatal consequences).

HOW TO TAKE CARE OF YOURSELF (WHILE REGAINING CONTROL OF YOUR CONCENTRATION AND FOCUS)

Obviously, the key to better focus and concentration is taking care of yourself. In this section, we will give you a short, easy to follow road map on how to place yourself on the right path. These steps are very simple to follow right from the start. But the important part is to stay consistent and stick with it as much as possible.

Here's what you need to do:

Get a good night's rest: Shoot for 7 to 9 hours of sleep per night. Power down your electronic devices including your smartphone at least 1 ½ to 2 hours prior to your scheduled bedtime (i.e.: If your bedtime is 10pm, do not use your electronic devices past 8:30 pm).

Reduce caffeine intake: Contrary to popular belief, caffeine may not be your saving grace when it comes to concentration. And it can also serve as a roadblock between you and a good night's sleep. If you do take in caffeine regularly, consider cutting it off at least six to eight hours before your scheduled bedtime (i.e. -- 2pm to 4pm if you go to bed at 10pm).

Switch up your eating habits: Instead of eating a few large meals per day, spread them out. Make them small and frequent. The more you eat, the more sluggish you might feel later on in the day. Also, you'll want to incorporate a good amount of fruits, veggies, whole grains, and lean proteins in your diet.

Reduce your stress levels: Stress can really do a number on your concentration. So, you'll need to find ways to go about reducing it even if you have limited time to yourself. Consider some brief meditation sessions. If you have enough time, you can read a book or write in a journal. In the event of the latter, write what's bothering you. Write about what you could have done differently throughout the day, so you are better prepared.

Just so we are clear, we don't want to overwhelm you with the idea of doing all these things at once. But you need to start somewhere. For example, if you want to get a good night's rest then start there. If you stay up late and want to go to bed earlier, you can gradually adjust the time week by week.

So, if you stay up until midnight and your goal is to go to bed at 10pm, start by going to bed an hour earlier one week. If that's a bit much, scale it back to a half hour instead. Scale it back by 30 to 60-minute increments per week until you reach the desired goal.

Remember, you want to make sure you still get seven to nine hours of sleep per night. And you want to know your cutoff times in terms of caffeine and using electronics. You'll be well-rested even if you follow a consistent sleep schedule.

THE LACK OF WILLPOWER, PERSEVERANCE, AND DEDICATION

In this section, we're going to talk about willpower, perseverance, and dedication. Each word will be defined and explained quickly in detail. It's important to have these three abilities on your journey towards self-discipline and mental toughness. Without them, the journey will be impossible to continue.

Willpower Defined And Explained

Willpower has multiple definitions. Yet, no matter what definition you read it will contain the same language. You will hear words like drive, self-control, self-discipline, and so on. Willpower is designed to help you restrain yourself from temptations (albeit for the short-term). The purpose is to ensure that you meet your long-term goals whatever they are.

If not for willpower, humanity would not have survived. Our ancestors had to rely on it in order to survive. We used it to hunt for food, take care of our families, and avoid any external threats to our livelihood. Now, here we are thousands of years later and it seems like it may not matter to most of us anymore.

The truth is that those with a higher level of willpower are usually happier, healthier, and able to manage stress in various situations. The question is: are we born with willpower or do we have to build on it like everything else? Believe it or not, the answer is yes...but to an extent.

Every person is born with willpower. And it can be built up like a muscle. If you are lacking in it, you can find ways to build on it and make it stronger. Like going to the gym, it will take time, commitment, and discipline to make it a complete success.

Willpower is also a test of patience and being able to restrain yourself. For example, let's take a look at an experiment known as the "Marshmallow Test". This was an experiment conducted by Walter Mischel, a psychologist at Columbia University.

Mischel administered the "Marshmallow Tests" to preschool aged children by placing a plate of marshmallows on the table. A child would sit at the table with the plate in front of them. Next, the child would be given the following instructions:

- The researcher administering the test told the child they would leave the room for a few minutes. If they waited for the researcher to return, they could take two marshmallows.
- If the child can't wait, they can ring the bell in front of them. Once the bell rings, the researcher will reappear and instruct them to take only one marshmallow.

Those who waited for the two marshmallows showed they had more willpower than the children that didn't. Years after the research was conducted, it was discovered that those with more willpower had higher SAT scores and a better body mass index (BMI).

The lack of willpower can lead to such links like poor academic performance and poor health. But it doesn't always have to be that way. You can reverse this just by building up on it.

Perseverance: What is it and how to use it

Perseverance is simply defined as doing the task at hand even if there are difficulties in the way. A prime example of this is when you are running a marathon and you are dealing with quite the headache. It makes you want to throw up and maybe even give up when you have a few miles left to go.

But you want to finish the race. You've trained for a year to get this far. So why let that all go to waste now? That is perseverance.

You have something planned out. But you know that there will be difficulties (and some surprises) along the way. It's important for you to be prepared and be able to tackle those obstacles so you can press on and finish the task.

If you are working on a group project, setbacks like people quitting (leading to being shorthanded) can happen. But it can be possible to get the job done with one less person (especially if they haven't pulled their weight).

When building up self-discipline and mental toughness, it will be a challenge right from the start. It will feel uncomfortable and rather painful. Because it's something that you are not used to on a daily basis. Remember, you'll also be making some sacrifices (but are worth the cost since they give you no "return on investment").

No matter how uncomfortable or "painful" it gets, you will want to press on. You've planned on attaining a goal and you took the initiative to start on it. If you've worked on it and make some progress, the last thing you want to do is wipe it all out just by quitting. Not only will it be a waste of time on your part, but it could be a waste of time for others (assuming it's a group project or goal you are working on).

When your back is against the wall and you have setback after setback, it's possible to achieve the task at hand no matter what. Your perseverance will set the stage towards disciplining yourself and developing a rock-hard mental toughness that will be hard to match. You are restraining yourself from taking the easy way out (and giving up).

Remember, giving up will have long term effects. One thing would be dwelling on the "what might have been". What if you didn't give up? What would happen if you did it differently?

Businessman (and two-time presidential candidate) Ross Perot said it best: "Most people give up when they're about to achieve success. They quit on the one-yard line. They give up at the last minute of the game, one foot from a winning touchdown."

In other words, perseverance will put you over the finish line. When you are tempted to give up despite everything thrown your way, don't do it. You may be a lot closer to achieving mental toughness and discipline than you realize.

Dedication: Why It Matters

Dedication is a synonym for commitment. To be dedicated to something, you are committed to getting the job done. You will settle for nothing less. When you are dedicated to something, you have an unmatched passion and loyalty to your mission, and you do not apologize for it.

Being dedicated to achieving discipline and mental toughness may be tough for most. But doing every little bit will put you a head above shoulders over those that don't do anything at all. All it takes for you is to take one step closer and you are miles ahead. However, it's important to not stop and resist the urge of quitting.

When it comes to developing mental toughness, it can be fueled by dedication. You could be dedicated to yourself or something that is a greater cause. Either way, it's important that you stay committed. You can develop mental toughness and stay dedicated even if you decide to take baby steps and not so many giant ones. As long as you take your time and stick to the plan, you're golden.

RECAP

The one person that stands in your way in terms of being more disciplined and mentally tough is you. It's important for you to plan and prioritize your day. The first thing you'll want to knock out are your most critical tasks. The sooner it's done, the better.

Don't worry about the tasks that are not so urgent or important. If a task is urgent, but doesn't hold a lot of importance, consider delegating the task to someone willing to get it done for you. Also, do not worry about the tasks that don't need to be done right away. There will come a time when you will take care of it. And last, don't do anything that will waste a lot of time (which can be otherwise invested in other things).

Overthinking can paralyze you. And it will lead you to not taking the necessary steps to achieve your goals. Figure out what's causing you to overthink. Come to the realization that there are things that will happen well beyond your control. If that happens, find a way to handle it to where it doesn't stress you.

It's true that we are no fans of responsibility. We find it easy to blame others for our mistakes and liabilities. Also, some of us tend to wait before someone else makes a move. That alone puts pressure on the other person to do something. Do your part and make the move. Others will follow. You don't have to be in a leadership position per se to take the initiative on something.

False hope syndrome is something that we are born with. But it can be curable. You cure it by setting goals (not resolutions). Outline them into steppingstones. And make sure they are in line with your values. Never let those values clash together or you may find yourself compromising one or the other.

Self-justification may be necessary, but it should be few. But you should never justify your mistakes, nor make an excuse for why you're procrastinating. Excuses are for the mentally weak and undisciplined.

Being a narcissist that carelessly hurts the morale of others while abusing the power of mental toughness will cast a dark shadow on you. And for most who travel down this path, it will be too late for them to turn back. Further proof that one person (i.e. -- themselves) is their own worst enemy.

It's important to own up to your mistakes and be able to move on early. Denying that you made a mistake and trying to justify it will make matters worse. Just move forward, accept your wrongdoing, and remind yourself not to do it again.

Finally, building discipline and mental toughness requires three things: willpower, perseverance, and dedication. They all go hand in hand. You were born with willpower. But it's what you do with it that will separate you among the others.

Perseverance will help you push through no matter how tough things get. And dedication to yourself or a higher cause will help you build the mental toughness that is needed to make perseverance a walk in the park.

A WORLD FULL OF DISTRACTIONS

I f there is one thing that is lurking on every corner no matter how near or far it is, it's danger. So, what's dangerous to someone's discipline and mental toughness? Distractions.

In today's modern world, distractions are all over the place. And we live right in the middle of it. Whether it's our smartphones, computers, or anything that is designed to get our attention, we tend to drop everything and pay even more attention to it.

Getting distracted will definitely fuel us to procrastinate more and focus on the less important things. Distractions have the power to "charm" us into how awesome it is to pay attention to them. It will get to the point where it lulls you into a trance and suddenly, you're hooked. Before you know it, hours have passed, and you still haven't done anything that needs to be done.

In this chapter, we'll be delving into distractions and how you can minimize them in your working environment. We'll also show you how to ensure that your relationship with others is helpful in your life and not the other way around. We'll also discuss the Hawthorne Effect and how you can use it to your advantage.

Let's tune in and get right to the chapter:

TAKE A GOOD LOOK AT EVERYTHING AROUND YOU

There's a potential distraction here. Another one there. A distraction across from you.

When you take a good look around you, there's a more than likely chance that there will be something that will distract you. Nine times out of ten, your phone might be within an arm's reach (so there's one potential distraction). Simply put, a distraction is defined as something designed to take your attention off the original task at hand so you can focus on the distraction itself.

Believe it or not, distractions exist in two types: external and internal. External distractions like your phone can be accessed at a moment's notice. On top of that, they can pop up out of nowhere whether it's three feet away or across the street.

Meanwhile, internal distractions will be all in your mind. You're stressed out, tired, or you have a thousand different things rushing through your head that you can't seem to quell. Dealing with these distractions will be a lot harder (but we'll show you how).

Simply put, distractions are all over the place. And the closest they can get to you is inside your mind. In other words, you'll never be too far away from one no matter where you are in the world. Distractions come in all different shapes, sizes, and forms.

Social media for example is a digital distraction. It can form in the shape that fits on your phone or computer screen. And there is all kinds of information that you can access from a social media platform alone. It deserves the top title of being the archenemy of discipline.

Social media may seem like it was designed for a greater good. For people to connect with friends and family. To keep informed about what's going on around them. The truth is that it winds up being one of the most ultimate distractions in existence.

Does it mean that you should get rid of social media period? It's your call. But it's a matter of limiting your use at times when you need to focus. When the task at hand needs a serious investment in time and attention, perhaps it's time to put away any distractions that may be within reach.

Believe it or not, excessive use of social media is not just a sign of being undisciplined. It also signals the possibility of depression and anxiety. The feeling of being wanted or appreciated. No, not everyone who uses social media is that way. But we can correlate social media use to not just a lack of discipline but also a lack of mental toughness.

One truth you might not realize is that our brains were made to distract us. Then again, you may not be surprised considering the fact we have already talked about internal distractions. You have things that run through your mind. The "what ifs" or the "should haves" are a good example. Also, the amount of information overloading in your brain will certainly distract you.

With all the information overload, you might end up opening up multiple tabs on your favorite web browser without thinking twice. And believe us when we say that this happens all the time. But if you can teach your brain to be less of a distraction and more of a weapon for positive thought and focus, only then it will serve you well in the long run.

CLEANSE YOUR WORK ENVIRONMENT OF DISTRACTIONS

In a work environment, distractions exist. As mentioned before, it doesn't matter where you are there's always going to be one closer than you think. It's important to consider cleansing your work area of these distractions as much as possible.

It may seem hard to do at first. But once you get the hang of it, it will be like second nature. In this section, we'll share with you our favorite tips on working more while getting less distracted. Distractions will be one of the major roadblocks towards discipline and mental toughness. With that in mind, here are some tips to consider:

Dispatch your technological distractions FIRST: With modern technology being one of the largest sources for many distractions, it's important that we start off with what we can do to minimize the distractions on our devices. If you are working on a computer, you should consider the idea of activating a blocker. There are plenty of blocking apps that you can run while you are in the process of working on something. You can use it to block social media apps and websites like Facebook or Twitter (if you use Google Chrome, there are some extensions that you can use like Cold Turkey). Don't think for a moment that your web browser is the only source for distraction. There's also your smartphone.

It's easy for us to take our phone out of our pockets the second we hear that notification sound go off. Before we know it, we're texting, commenting, tweeting, and so on. One of the things you should do is put the phone on airplane mode or "do not disturb" mode. This will allow your phone to stifle any notifications for as long as it's activated. One more thing you need to do is place your phone in a different part of the room.

If your workspace is inside your house, put it in a different room like a living room or kitchen. If you're in an office setting, put it in a locker or a filing cabinet near you (preferably in one of the cabinets with a lock. Just make sure you have the key before you accidentally lock it and can't get to it).

Focus on your most time sensitive and critical tasks first: Your most time-sensitive and critical tasks must be done as soon as possible. Failure to do so will lead to quite a bit of chaos. Not to mention, these tasks can be hard to do when the pressure is on and timing is not in your favor. You should focus on the first two or three critical tasks of the day first before doing anything else. One critical task may also be enough before moving on to the others. Either way, the more you get out of the way the better.

Use minimums to your advantage: What would you do? 50 pushups a day or 5? If you answered 5, good choice. Doing the minimum amount of work rather than focus on something larger will help you get in the mindset of doing little but ending up going a little beyond that. So, if the goal is 5 pushups, you may feel inclined to do more work. From there on, you'll be able to up your minimums to a point where you can do a bit more without breaking a sweat (or your mind). The minimum is a baby step closer to the ultimate goal. Do the minimal amount, take a break, then do it again.

Eliminate any sources of internal distractions: Internal distractions can and will occur at any time. You could be stressed. You could be tired. Or maybe even both. The solutions we provide are probably some you've heard of before. Get a good night's rest the night before. Meditate for five minutes before you begin the day's work. Anything that can be proven to minimize stress can work to your advantage. Just remember, internal distractions are just as bad as the external ones. If you can't get rid of them outright, find ways to minimize them as best you can.

Run a visualization through your head: Before every big game, an athlete will visualize their success. Nine times out of ten, it works to perfection. You can do this yourself. Imagine yourself working on the tasks at hand without stress or with the feeling that nothing can stop you. Take a few minutes to ponder on it. If you can visualize it, it can certainly give you the confidence to get it done. Another visualization technique is to reverse engineer your accomplishment. In other words, start backwards from the end to the beginning. Visualize your actions in small steps.

Minimize external distractions: This one might be a lot easier than dealing with the internal distractions. This could mean moving to a quieter area, putting on headphones with your favorite music or binaural beats, or just putting away your phone or devices. The more external distractions you can identify, the better. Find ways to minimize them or temporarily eliminate them until the work is done.

Keep the momentum going: When you have all your distractions tuned out, you'll have a clear path to accomplishing the task at hand. You work at least on the bare minimum, take a quick break, and repeat. It's all about focusing on that one thing, putting the pedal to the medal and never looking back. Distraction can be a momentum killer. Just remember to focus on the small things, nothing too big and crazy.

YOUR RELATIONSHIP WITH OTHERS SHOULD HELP YOU, NOT SABOTAGE YOU

Relationships in your life are not a burden to you and your goals. So, they shouldn't be considered an outright distraction. However, there is work to be done. So how do you go about achieving your goals and minimizing distractions without upsetting those who are most important to you?

We can sum this up in one word: communication. There is no such thing as the perfect work/life balance. There are days when the workday can require you to put in extra time. Will it cut into time that will otherwise be spent on your significant other or family? Unfortunately, yes. But the good news is it's a lot less than you think.

Family will always come first no matter what. This is something you want to reiterate with them when you are communicating with them. If there is some kind of major project coming up where it requires your time and attention, you need to make them aware of it. Let them know that there will be times when you'll be home late and there may be limited time you can spend with anyone (since you're going to need your rest).

Tell them that you are not ignoring them (nor forgetting about them). After all, let your family know that they are the reason why you have the drive to work hard. The most important people in your life are your best cheerleaders. They inspire you to better yourself when others will not. Even if no one else will support you, they will. They are your closest allies when the going gets tough.

When relationships become distractions

Another thing you want to do is evaluate your relationships outside of your family. Are most of the people that you associate yourself with more positive or negative? If you are dealing with negative people in your life, they will end up being a distraction. Lucky for you, you'll have a good idea of keeping that distraction at bay. You can give them less attention or cut them out completely if they are too toxic.

Those who understand what your line of work is and the important things you need to focus on will likely develop a positive relationship with you. They see distraction as a negative thing and will respect your privacy when you need it. Neediness is a distraction within itself. Plus, it's also a two-way street.

For example, someone will need to see you or talk to you. And there are those who need to communicate with someone because they are unhappy, alone, or what have you. Neediness is something you can't deal with or have in your life. When relationships become distractions, the first thing you need to do is minimize it as much as possible. If it gets too bad, cutting out the distractions without thinking twice is something you can do without shame.

Building your support system is key

When focusing on tasks that need to be completed, it's good to have a support system in place. People like your family and friends should be a part of it. However, they need to realize that when things get busy, they will give you their full-throated support and leave it at that so you can focus. They won't bother you nor will they doubt you in getting the job done.

A support system doesn't have to be ridiculously large. You can build it with a few like-minded friends, and it can be stronger than steel. Don't be afraid to reach out to people that you want to be a part of it either. It's good to vet people who you want as your most trusted allies. Plus, it can be a tough, but rewarding task.

Strengthen and maintain your relationships

Relationships are a two-way street. One person does their part to keep it strong and well maintained. You return the favor (and vice versa). It can't be where one person is solely responsible for building it. Remember, communication is the key to a strong and healthy relationship. Without it, there's nothing that either party will bring to the table.

One more thing, aside from regular communication you want to build the relationship by building value while expecting nothing in return. If you try to grovel or the like, then people will be well aware of ulterior motives you might have.

USE THE HAWTHORNE EFFECT TO YOUR ADVANTAGE

Next, we'll be discussing what is known as the Hawthorne Effect. What exactly is it? It's named after an experiment that was conducted almost a hundred years ago. It was believed that when someone was being watched or the central part of someone's focus, they would perform their tasks (and with great effectiveness). It's almost as if they don't want them to fail in front of anyone.

While someone might not literally be watching you while you work, you want to act as if someone is watching your every move. Your boss will always keep tabs on employees who are hired to do the work. If you deliver the work as expected, then you are rewarded. If you do nothing, your boss will notice that you are not pulling your weight. You may be reprimanded or terminated from your job.

If you are part of a group project, you are being watched for doing your part. Rest assured, everyone in your group is watching each other so everyone is on the same page and fulfills their responsibilities. If it's in a school setting, they know that the grade they get as a group will either benefit or hinder their overall economic performance.

People perform better and will get the task done if they know they are being watched. For example, there was one research experiment done where medical staffers were the subject. When watched, the staffers were 55 percent more likely to wash their hands and comply with safety precautions compared to those not being watched.

As mentioned, it's easy to make mistakes and do little work when you are not being watched. Just because you're not being watched all the time, it doesn't mean that you should slack off. There will come a time when you may be subject to some kind of random accountability check. It's important to follow deadlines and get the most important tasks done at every opportunity you have. You'll want to approach each task as if you will be evaluated on it after completion.

The Hawthorne Effect will make it so that accountability partners are much needed than ever. That way, you hold each other accountable for whatever tasks you may perform. The lack of accountability can lead to a decline in productivity not just for yourself but also your partner. It's important to find someone you can trust to hold you accountable while they do their own part.

ENHANCE YOUR FOCUS AND UNPLUG REALITY

In a world full of distractions, it is absolutely paramount to make sure that your focus is better than ever. Sometimes, it's always a good idea to disconnect yourself from reality for a few hours just so you can focus. One of the best ways to go about increasing your focus is going on a digital detox.

A digital detox is defined as pulling yourself away from social media or even digital devices. This can be done every day simply by not hopping on social media or looking at your phone for a few hours. Some will even take on the challenge of going without social media for days, weeks, or even months. It all comes down to willpower.

THE BENEFITS OF A DIGITAL DETOX

If you have never done a digital detox, then you may want to consider doing one. Below is a list of benefits that you may enjoy should you go forward with the idea. A lot of people try to do one but quickly give up (a recurring theme for most of us). And it goes back to the value of feeling connected to other people. However, there is a benefit that will make you feel more connected to the people you appreciate even more.

Let's take a look at the list of benefits now:

1. Improved connection with other people

It's no secret that cell phone use can be a burden on human interaction. At least 82 percent of Americans will share that sentiment. That's why it's always a good idea to keep your phone in your pocket and on vibrate while you are spending quality time with family or with your friends. It's a lot better to have a fulfilling conversation or have a ton of fun without the use of any digital devices.

The last thing you want to do is dig out your phone while talking to the other person. The latter will feel ignored. They will feel like they don't provide you with enough personal value. Sometimes, there may be that piece of information stuck in your head where you subconsciously dig out your phone to look it up without even thinking.

Instead of looking it up mindlessly, you can mention bringing it up in the form of a question during your conversation (if you feel that it's relevant). If not, make a mental note to look it up online later.

2. Reduces stress

Did you know that technology is a source of stress? Yep. Technology can go haywire or someone may say something on the Internet that is outright ridiculous. Either way, something about technology will stress someone out. It's important for you to refrain from long-term use. The person who spends an hour a day on their phone will be less stressed than someone who spends a few hours per day.

3. You'll sleep better

Electronics emit a blue light that can reduce natural melatonin levels. Melatonin is a chemical that helps you sleep at night. That's why it is important to shut down any electronics at least an hour and a half or two hours prior to bedtime (as we've mentioned early on in the book). Not only does better rest help you sleep, but it's also a building block in reducing amounts of stress. Better sleep and a digital detox go hand in hand. The next benefit will explain why.

4. Better focus and concentration

A good night's rest and a digital detox will give you a better chance at having more focus and concentration throughout the day. You don't feel distracted in the slightest. Also, your attention span will increase four seconds in length compared to the average person. Believe it or not, the average person's attention span is a mere eight seconds. To have a twelve second attention span will set you a head above shoulders over the rest.

5. Increased problem-solving skills

When there's a problem and the digital distractions are not consuming you whole, you will be more alert and aware of the problem. And it will also help you use your brain by thinking a little deeper. It will also help you recall things better than those who have to rely on modern technology.

6. You'll be a lot happier

It's widely known that those who are highly dependent on social media and technology will likely have some kind of depression. But a digital detox for a few hours or even long-term (days or weeks) can improve your happiness considerably. You will be able to have a vested interest in doing activities that you'll enjoy more. Not to mention, they will be a bit more focused on that task rather than retreating back to their digital device.

Logging off social media and the Internet in general will more than likely improve your level of happiness (even for the long-term). On top of that, your levels of anxiety will be reduced considerably.

HOW TO DO A DIGITAL DETOX

Now that you know the benefits of doing a digital detox, perhaps it's time for you to try it out for yourself. Not only will it be a test of your discipline and mental toughness, but it will give you an opportunity to iron some of life's wrinkles. You may figure out why you're stressed or feeling less than happy in terms of your overall mood. So, with that in mind, let's take a look at some tips that you'll need to take to heart when planning to do a digital detox:

Determine how much time you want to spend: Do you want to go without technology for a few hours a day? Or do you want to go longer? This will depend on how severe the need is. If you're looking at your phone every few minutes and placing a high importance on every notification, you know it's time for a digital detox. To start, you would want to consider starting off slow (about 4 to 6 hours a day) and then gradually working your way up. Once you become comfortable with the idea of going without your devices for longer periods, you can make the adjustments.

Consider alternative activities: What do you want to do instead of looking at your phone? Think about the activities you enjoy doing. Ask yourself, what would you do if you didn't have your phone on hand. Would you read a book? Why not take a walk outdoors?

Consider a cut off time and stick with it: For those who want to do a more scaled back version of a digital detox, it's important to choose a time where you "can't touch" your phone. One prime example is at least an hour and a half to two hours prior to your scheduled bedtime (something we've touched on earlier in the book). When that time comes, you honor that cut off time. Not a second longer.

Shut off notifications: Take a look at the apps that you normally use. There's a pretty good chance that most of your notifications are from your social media apps (Facebook, Twitter, Instagram, etc.). You can shut them off completely or during work hours. Either way, it will work to your advantage.

Say "no" to apps for a week: One of the key aspects of self-discipline is being able to say "no" to things that may be hard to resist. Clearly, your most used apps like social media is one of them. If they are the apps you are planning to shut off for the week, make sure that your friends and family have other alternative forms of contacting you (like phone or email).

Clean out your inbox: How many email newsletters do you subscribe to? We have a habit of letting in so many into our inbox. You have one email in your inbox. Then it goes to ten. Then a hundred. It's so overwhelming you're just trying to keep up. If you're getting pummeled with newsletters and such over the course of the day, your inbox is in need of some serious cleaning. Unsubscribe from email lists that provide no value to you. If they are from an online store you haven't shopped at in the past 60 to 90 days and have no plans to buy there again, unsub from the list.

These are the tips that you want to follow when you want to do a digital detox. It may be hard to say no to your favorite apps for at least a week. And it might be tough to keep away from your phone during the most important hours of the day.

A digital detox is one of the true tests for discipline, willpower, commitment, and most importantly mental toughness. Think of this as the brand-new marshmallow test. Except, you're not waiting on someone to come back. Waiting one week to access Facebook or Instagram again is the challenge.

It will also help you find alternative things to do so your mind is more focused on that than the desire to hop on your phone and post something. Just take it one day at a time and don't focus on the week itself. Start out small and minimal.

RECAP

It's true that the world is full of distractions. Unfortunately, they will still exist all over the place both around you and inside your head. The only thing you can do is minimize them as much as possible.

Your external distractions can be minimized by working in a much quieter area where you are allowed to maximize your focus. Tune out as much of the outside noise as you can. These can be as easy as slapping on a pair of headphones, shutting off your notifications between a specific time period, and being able to program your computer to deny you access to certain websites throughout a period of the day.

Internal distractions also exist. They may be tough to minimize them (not to mention, they will take time). The best ways to deal with them are getting a good night's rest and reducing stress. Believe it or not, there is a solution where you're allowed to do both things (and it's all linked to your use of electronic devices).

It's important for you to stay the course, keep building momentum, and never lose focus. One instance of breaking momentum and you'll fall behind. If you need to take a break, take a five to ten-minute break and prevent using your electronic devices (for obvious reasons).

Your relationships will matter most. They shouldn't be treated like a burden either. These people in your life are your family, close friends, and colleagues. It's true that you need some alone time to focus on your work. But sometimes, you need to be aware that you have a support group consisting of individuals that are all rooting for you.

If anything, they are here to help you push through and hold yourself accountable. Speaking of accountability, that's where the Hawthorne Effect comes into play. You won't have someone watching over you all the time. But those who know of what you can accomplish will be interested in how things are going. Act as if someone is keeping a watchful eye on you at all times (without feeling paranoid).

Lastly, it never hurts to unplug. Doing a digital detox for a short or long-term period can work to your advantage. Not only will you be less distracted, but you'll also find yourself more in tune with your mind. You'll feel happier, more productive, and see things at a different angle compared to most people.

III

UNEARTHING YOUR REASON
TO CHANGE

START WITH THE WAY YOU THINK

Most of the challenges you will face in your life will focus more on the mental aspect versus the physical. In sports, they say most of it is 90 percent mental while the physical part is only 10 percent. When it comes to discipline and mental toughness, the same concept pretty much applies.

In this chapter, we'll focus on one part of the mental side of things. It starts with the way you think. It's up to you to adopt a mindset that will allow you to go from undisciplined to disciplined (and mentally weak to tough). We'll define what mindset is and discuss the two types that exist: fixed and growth.

A bit of a spoiler alert: the fixed mindset isn't going to be what you'll want to adopt here. Therefore, we'll be talking about how to adopt the growth mindset and how you'll use it to your advantage on the journey towards being the most disciplined, mentally tough individual on the planet.

If you are looking for a way to bust through the mental blocks but don't know how, this chapter will help you take a wrecking ball to them so you can press on. Let's jump right in and start with the definition of mindset:

Mindset: A way of thinking or a frame of mind.

Yes, the definition is simple and to the point. Don't we wish that switching to a positive mindset was as simple as that? There are two types of mindsets that exist. Let's take a look at them and explain how they work:

Fixed mindset: This kind of mindset is where nothing seems to change. The qualities of which you possess are unchangeable and you're stuck with it forever. However, that's just the definition. But it's possible to change it.

Growth mindset: With this mindset, you can be able to go forward each day with the belief that you can improve and grow. You can grow and strengthen yourself through hard work and dedication. This is the mindset we want you, dear reader, to aim for. Is it impossible to acquire? Only if you think that way.

With a fixed mindset, there's always the fear of being judged and worrying about not living up to someone's expectations. Those with a growth mindset don't care who's judging them. And they could care less about who's expectations they live up to (or don't live up to). If anything, they are focused on the goals they set forth and move forward.

Those with a fixed mindset and a growth mindset are susceptible to making mistakes. Yet, the only difference is they handle them in a different way. Those with a fixed mindset find mistakes to be the "devil's work". So, they try to avoid them like the plague. And it is for this reason they try to become perfectionists. And if you know a perfectionist or two, you notice that they share the common emotion of getting angry when things are less than perfect.

Those with a fixed mindset find mistakes to be a "be all end all thing". And thus, failure means the end of the world. They don't learn from their mistakes and don't bother to take on any other challenges for fear that it would be too tough and complex (thus the fear of failure settles in quickly).

A growth mindset sees things a different way. They know that mistakes happen. They take them as learning lessons, so they don't make the same mistakes again. They don't care about perfection, but they will never settle for anything less than satisfactory. They know that quality matters most in what they do. But as long as they get the task done, they should have no problem.

YOUR MINDSET CAN DICTATE YOUR NEXT WORDS AND ACTIONS

If you think it's hard to tell who has a fixed mindset and who has one that is growth oriented, you may be surprised. In fact, you can hear it in their voice or language. You can see it in their body language if you are very observant. You don't have to be an expert at reading people to know what kind of mindset another person has.

Yet, you'd be hard-pressed to find someone who has more of a growth mindset. Especially, when they have goals that they know they can achieve no matter how long it takes them. But that doesn't mean they are few and far between in the slightest.

You can adopt a mindset of growth if you so choose to do so. And when you do, you'll find yourself speaking in a different way. Instead of saying "I can't", say "I can". Or instead of "if I fail, it's over" you can say "if I fail, I'll learn from it and be ready for next time". It's hard to understand why it's difficult for someone to switch their mindset from fixed to growth.

They say, "fake it until you make it". This may work to your advantage to an extent. Or you can act as if you have already achieved your goal. When you act as if you've accomplished something, you'll feel like you can accomplish the next task with ease. It just might help you on your journey towards adopting a growth mindset.

But one thing to keep in mind is to be congruent. If you are acting that you have a growth mindset but react to something negative in a way someone with a fixed mindset would, then it might be hard to gain trust from people if you seem to be putting up some kind of front. However, you'll want to act as if someone is watching your every move (hello Hawthorne, we meet again).

This means you'll need to push yourself to weather through that negativity. You have no other choice. People are watching and assuming that you have a good mindset. Don't prove them wrong or fool them into thinking otherwise. Not only will it force you into a situation where you can level up on discipline and mental toughness, but you'll soon realize that adopting a growth mindset isn't so bad after all.

THE MINDSET OF A DISCIPLINED AND MENTALLY TOUGH PERSON

So, what exactly does the mindset of a disciplined and mentally tough person look like? In this section, we'll give you an in-depth look. Obviously, they have a growth mindset. But what specifically goes through the mind of someone who is already disciplined and mentally tough? Learn from this section and take notes so you can be able to reverse engineer exactly how to adopt that very mindset from the end to beginning.

A disciplined and mentally tough person is more than likely to embrace challenges whenever they are thrown at them. They know that failure isn't the be all to end all. They are aware of the potential setbacks that can occur. But they are ready for them at any given moment. Once they complete tasks, they are not afraid to receive positive criticism that will better them in the future.

They don't care about the "negative", unsolicited criticism some people tend to give out to make the latter feel bad. A disciplined and mentally tough person will learn from pieces of advice from their mentors before applying it in the future. Depending on their goals, they take a look at people who have already achieved them. They study what they've done, what their setbacks were, and how they overcame them.

They learn the stories about someone's success, and they use it as inspiration to push themselves forward. Now they know who to model their success after, they tailor it to their own approach towards their goals and accomplishments. They know they can achieve a higher level of results. They don't care how long it will take them.

If they achieve it in a short amount of time, good. If it takes a bit longer than average, they'll just shrug it off. At least they got it done and that's all that matters. They will say they had setbacks, but they managed to get through them. They have the determination to push through anything that gets in the way.

Lastly, they know that a lapse in discipline can occur (and yes, it does happen). But when they recognize it, they pick themselves back up and get back on the path. They hold themselves accountable and get straight to work. The Dali Lama said it best:

"A disciplined mind leads to happiness. An undisciplined mind leads to suffering."

— THE DALI LAMA

Those words could not be spoken more truthfully. However, it's hard to adopt since they seem to have the desire to stay ahead and push anyone who stands in the way. However, a disciplined person knows that competition is not their worst enemy. They see a competitor as someone who could be of value to them at some point down the road.

Someone who is self-disciplined enough will stick to the plan. They will stay focused and not make any changes to "keep up" with someone. The whole "keeping up with the Joneses" attitude is a trait of those who are undisciplined. And that alone could lead them to an unhappy life, financial distress, and so on. A mentally disciplined individual doesn't worry about people who have the best things and flaunt them.

Discipline and mental toughness are two things that will help you achieve the best level of happiness. It is your weapon against those who try to buy nice things in order to cover for their insecurities (meanwhile, while triggering the other people to do the same and thus continuing a vicious cycle). Don't fall for the trap of "keeping up" because someone else decides to compensate for their lack of confidence and security.

OVERCOMING THE FEAR WITHIN

Fear is another thing that holds us back from doing anything. Yet, for the person that adopts the growth mindset they know that fear is something that doesn't faze them in the slightest. They are afraid of things going south or some kind of setback. But they just say, "screw it" and get on with the task. Fear will hold you back if you let it.

You will fail. You will feel like crap. But the way you handle it will set you ahead of the others. You may feel embarrassed. But it gives you the energy to learn from your mistakes and move forward. Don't think for a moment that the people who love you most (and are a part of your support system) will lose faith in you if you screw up. It's not like they expect you to get it perfect on the first try.

If anything, fear should be fuel. It should be that energy and drive that will push you to get the work done and earn the reward that is the sense of accomplishment you feel after the fact. Yes, fear is a powerful emotion. But you can be able to convert it into something that will drive you out of your comfort zone and do something different. When you're in your comfort zone, things will be the same old, mundane, boring things. And that will really make you feel like you've done nothing with your life.

Too much comfort and complacency will cause you to miss out on the things that matter most. Meanwhile, if you have a willingness to face fear and stand outside of your comfort zone then there is no sense of waiting for the right moment. That moment to get something done is right now. Restrain yourself from doing what otherwise could be the exact opposite (like doing nothing).

TIPS ON HOW TO HANDLE FEAR

Below is a list of things that you can do in order to handle your fear. This will give you an opportunity to get to know yourself on a much deeper level. You may have some fears that you never knew about. Or you may be afraid of a lesser number of things. Either way, it is important to know your fears and find a way to conquer them.

Here are the following tips to put to good use:

Write down what you're afraid of: First thing you should do is get a piece of paper. Or open up a word document if you feel more comfortable. Spend time thinking about what you're afraid of. The deeper you go into detail, the better. What are your fears? Why are you afraid of it? What can do you to face that fear or at least stop it from getting the best of you?

Realize that you're in control: As the old saying goes, "those who control you, have the power over you". Do you want to live your life knowing that your every fear will control the frame? Or do you want to gain control over fear and use it to your advantage? Letting fear control, you will lead to inaction. And inaction means getting nothing accomplished.

Adopt positive affirmations: Affirmations are a great way to mentally program yourself into what you should believe in. As silly as it may sound, it has actually worked for people. You can say things like "I will not let my fear control me" a few times while looking at yourself in the mirror. You should consider putting affirmations to good use on a regular basis. You can do them in the morning the first thing you wake up and do them again before you go to bed. Either way, they will be helpful in developing your mental toughness.

Visualize yourself facing fear: As mentioned in the book, we suggested visualizing your accomplishment. Another reason why we are so big on it is because we see ourselves getting the job done without fear controlling us. And we imagine ourselves enjoying that sense of accomplishment that rushes through our veins. That feeling can become reality if we say, "to hell with fear", put the pedal to the medal, and get to work. It's better to visualize your accomplishments before getting started rather than visualize about what might have been.

It's okay to talk about them: Your fears aren't something that people will laugh at. If they do, it's more of their problem than it is yours. Talk to someone who you can trust like a member of your family or a trusted friend (especially someone in your support system). Tell them what your plans are and why you're not acting on them due to a certain fear. There's a good chance that they will reassure you that everything will be fine. If you succeed, great. If you fail, don't let it get to you. Opportunities will arise (even if they sound like some kind of once in a lifetime thing).

These tips will help you overcome your fear of whatever it is that may be holding you back from doing anything. Don't let fear restrain you. It should be the exact opposite (which is pretty much one of the main points of this book).

VISUALIZING THE FUTURE AHEAD OF YOU

As mentioned before, visualization will play a huge role in helping you press through fear so you can accomplish your goals. It will also help you along the path towards self-discipline and being able to toughen up mentally. Visualizing the steps you take and the outcome you want to achieve is essential.

How do you go about visualizing your success? What can you do to ensure that things will work to your advantage? We'll be taking a look at some tips below on how you can visualize your success for both the short-term and long-term.

Before we go forward with the tips, it's important to set this one condition: **you need to know what you want.** What is your ultimate goal? What is it exactly that you want?

Without a clear goal in mind, you won't be able to visualize it and be able to go forward in achieving it. Not to mention, you won't have the ability to have the discipline or the mental toughness to make it happen.

Here are some suggestions that we consider effective:

Put together a vision board: Vision boards have grown in popularity over the years. The way these work are as follows: you have a cork board or poster that you can create into a makeshift collage. These are quite inexpensive to put together. And if you see an image that reminds you of your goal, you can always add it onto your vision board. Just one more reminder why the goal you set to achieve is important.

Write in a gratitude journal: A journal is a great way to visualize and write down what you are thankful for. At night, think of five to ten things you are grateful for. You can also write down something about what's been bothering you as of late, what you could have done differently today, and plan for the future so that you are mentally prepared and ready to take on the next phase of your goal.

Meditation: Of course, meditation will work to your advantage if you are looking to change the way you think. Not only will meditation put you in that "in the moment" mindset. But it will also help you bear down and focus on what you need to accomplish. Before you know it, you'll be done with your most critical tasks with a little more time to spare.

Write a "dream check": While it sounds a bit crazy, you can write a "dream check" of an amount of money you want to shoot for in your lifetime. One of the famous examples of this method was done by none other than actor Jim Carrey. Before rising to stardom, he wrote himself a check for $10 million. He dated it for Thanksgiving 1995. He used it as a visualization tool, and it helped him become one of the best comedic actors in the world. Believe it or not, he landed a role that earned him $10 million by Thanksgiving 1995. The point of this is you can write yourself out a "check" for a monetary value that you realistically want to achieve. Put it on your wall and use it as a source to drive you to perform the tasks and goals that you need to get there.

RECAP

Mental blocks can deter you from changing your mindset or serve as some kind of obstacle that you can blow past. Your mindset can change. It is up to you to determine whether or not you have a fixed mindset or one where growth and improvement is possible. The reality is that most people may not be able to make the switch. But if you decide to go from fixed to growth in terms of mindset, you'll be ahead of a lot of people.

It's important to know the mindset of someone who is disciplined and mentally tough. They carry themselves in such a way that it shows in their body language, the way they say things, and how they deal with stress. One way to familiarize yourself with the mindset of a disciplined and mentally tough individual is to reverse engineer what they have done. Start from the end and finish at the beginning. You'll know this mindset backwards and forwards and know how to take the necessary steps to get where you need to be.

Fear will become a mental block that you'll need to bust through as well. It should be viewed as fuel for pressing on and moving forward no matter what the outcome is. It's fine to visualize a positive outcome in the beginning. But it's important to not think too much of it and just focus on getting a certain task done. If the outcome is not what you desired, take a moment to learn about what went wrong and consider the steps you need to take so you can prevent another mistake.

Visualizing the future is a tool that will instill confidence, discipline, and mental toughness. We know what each of us wants. To incorporate the emotions of our visualizations will help us become more effective in our tasks and help us handle stress and adversity wherever it pops up.

Consider the idea of incorporating visualization tools that will help you push you to become more disciplined, mentally tough, and someone who will rise to the challenge and conquer it. Your mind can be a dangerous weapon against adversity and setbacks. Or it can cave under pressure. Either way, it's up to you to make the mindset change to determine what will happen in those situations.

ENGINEERING A DISCIPLINED LIFE

A disciplined life is filled with rewards. One of them is the ongoing sense of accomplishment. The fact that you can get the job done without the setbacks and obstacles getting to you can be quite the feeling. This can be you. And if you want that, keep reading this chapter.

In this chapter, we'll be talking about the "new normal" and how you should embrace it going forward. We'll also take a look at how discipline is like a child. Something that you can "birth" and nurture into something that will be a part of you for the rest of your living days. We'll also talk about what a life of a disciplined person looks like.

The nurturing part of discipline will be very important. So, we'll show you how to connect yourself with the right kind of people who share the same mindset and discipline as you do. And lastly, we'll talk about how you should take the proactive approach to ensure that you are a disciplined individual from the morning you get out of bed to the moment you hit your head on the pillow for a good night's rest.

Onward.

EMBRACING YOUR NEW NORMAL

The words "new normal" have been a part of our vocabulary as of late. Especially with the COVID-19 pandemic changing the ball game on how we live, how we do business, and so on. Some of the things we've considered normal have been unceremoniously thrown out the window without warning. Things that could have been possible in a few years' time have now become the "normal" thing to do.

As a mentally tough and disciplined person, the best thing to do is accept and adapt to change. Even in our lifetime, we may need to change the way we live because we have no choice but to do so. For example, you might be a sucker for spicy foods. But you have a health condition that will discourage you from enjoying them. By order of your doctor, you can't have as much as you used to (or never again).

The new normal may seem like a shock to the system to so many. And many will continue asking questions and have few answers to work with. To a disciplined individual, they are nervous about the new normal. But they get through it with a smile on their face knowing that they can take on the challenge. The uncertainty of what's on the other end makes it even more enticing for them to continue forward.

This new normal will be a challenge to many. Those who rise above it will come out on top. Will you be one of them?

GIVING BIRTH TO DISCIPLINE

Discipline is like a child. You give "birth" to it and raise it as your own. It should be a part of your life. A child needs to be well taken care of so it can grow to be strong both in mind and body. The same can be said for your discipline. It should not be abused or neglected in any way. This is how you should view discipline from this point forward. It's important for you to nurture your discipline and watch it grow into something that will make you even tougher mentally and a better person overall.

Is raising a child an easy task? If you're a parent, you already know the answer. It's not as easy as people think. But the rewards are sweet. Your discipline may not be easy to maintain and nurture. But imagine the kind of benefits and rewards you reap in the process. What may seem like a harmless task that you're doing (like procrastinating), it's hurting your discipline in more ways than one.

Being able to discipline yourself and nurturing it will help make things easy to do. You can develop a new skill with ease. You can get the most critical tasks done with more time to spare. You can resist the urge to get sucked into things that are actually a waste of your time. If you let setbacks get to you or get engaged in "time sucking" activities, your discipline will suffer.

The "Motivation" Myth

People say that you should do a certain task when you feel "motivated" enough. The problem is motivation is elusive. If you look for it, it will go in the opposite direction. Most people are mentally focused on searching for it and forgetting about the tasks before them. Before they know it, they waste plenty of time.

If you want to improve your writing, some advise you to work on it whenever you feel motivated. Why not write anyways? Perhaps write a hundred words first thing in the morning. Then the following day, you can up it to about two hundred and work your way up.

The same can be said about losing weight. Why work out if you have the "spare time"? You know you have a block of time that you can carve out and dedicate it to working out regularly. A few days out of the week for an hour might be just what you need. Just find that available time slot and dedicate it to working out.

Lastly, if you are serious about saving money then consider setting aside a specific amount of money each time you earn. In George Clason's "The Richest Man In Babylon", one of the rules is to set aside 10 percent of what you earn. Just take that portion and set it off to the side in a safe or a box. Use it in case of emergencies, not when you want to splurge (another test in willpower and discipline, now that we think about it).

If you need something to get you going, visualization is the key. Circling back to our previous chapter, you can imagine yourself in your ideal situation and instill the emotions that will drive you to get the job done. Visualization is a hell of a lot better than trying to locate that ever elusive motivation, don't you think?

LOOKING AT THE LIFE OF DISCIPLINED PEOPLE

In the previous chapter, we gave you an in-depth look of the mindset of mentally tough people. Now, we'll be taking a glimpse at the life of someone who lives a disciplined life. And we don't have to go too far in depth by discovering the kind of traits they possess. You can tell who is disciplined and who is not by the way they act and how they go about their day.

We will go over a list of these traits, so you have a good idea of what to expect while you are in the beginning stages of being more disciplined yourself. Once you start adopting these traits, it will show. You won't have to say a single word to declare that you are self-disciplined. These are the traits that you'll likely develop over time:

Resisting temptation: Obviously, temptation is the enemy of discipline. No matter how hard you want to give into it, you know that within yourself is the power to control yourself. Temptation can be powerful only if you allow it to happen. Temptation comes at the worst times (like emotional low points). As long as you are aware of its presence and decide not to give in, you're in the driver's seat.

Endless commitment: Those who are disciplined and committed speak their words and stick to it. When they declare a goal that they want to accomplish, they stick with it. Period. End of story. When you say it to other people, some of them may keep a watchful eye on you. So, when they ask you how it's going, how will you respond? With shock and aghast? Or with confidence knowing that you got it done.

They take good care of themselves: A person who takes care of themselves is not only disciplined, but they also have a high level of self-respect that can't be matched. They take care of themselves mentally and physically and do it with a plan in place every day.

They set limits and boundaries: A disciplined person knows their limits and their boundaries. They set them and never go beyond them. In other words, they say no to things easily. They don't want to cross a line they set for themselves. Limits and boundaries are a true test for discipline. Keep within them and you will certainly pass.

Emotions are second to them: When it comes to taking action, their emotions take a backseat (and rightfully so). Whenever there is a goal or a task that needs to be done, they do it anyways even if they don't feel like doing it. The task of overriding your emotions and performing a routine task can be difficult for most people. Thus, doing so will lead to procrastination.

They set a deadline and meet it: You have a goal to achieve and want to meet it in six months. No "pushing it back". No "rescheduling". No nothing. They stick with the deadline and keep at it until that day (or before that). Is it fine to complete the task ahead of schedule? You bet. You must resist the urge to procrastinate or wait for a time where motivation appears to get the tasks done.

The prize is the focus: There are plenty of words that you can conjure up in the English language that will be a nugget of truth. "Keep your eye on the prize" is one of them. Whether you have a setback or two or fell off the wagon and haven't gotten anything done in days, knowing what the end reward is and focusing on it is key.

You will soon remember that you have a goal to accomplish and you'll do whatever it takes to get it done regardless of what's getting in the way.

They focus on the small things: When it comes to achieving a bigger goal, they know that it comes down to focus on the small things. They break up the much larger goal into little pieces. Think of it like a music album. You can't just record one song and call it good. You can record ten of them and have a hit album that your fans will love. One song equals a step towards achieving your much larger goal. The same can be said about a book. Write a thousand words and you are closer to getting the entire thing done. Get the idea?

MAKE FRIENDS WITH PEOPLE WHO ARE SMARTER THAN YOU

There's an old saying: "If you are the smartest person in the room, find another room where you are not". Not only will this help you build more discipline and mental toughness, it will humble you in the fact that there may be someone who is more disciplined than you, smarter than you, and has accomplished more. Don't let this be a personal indictment against you. These people are not your enemies. They are people you can learn from and inspire you to be your best self.

Now, the question is: how will you surround yourself with people smarter than you? Supplementally, where exactly can you find them? The answer may seem like something you might not expect, but people who are smarter than you can be found just about anywhere. It's a matter of knowing how to spot them.

SIGNS THAT SOMEONE IS SMARTER THAN YOU

It's not that there is a specific place where you can find people smarter than you (aside from maybe a local MENSA chapter meeting). Being observant is key when seeking out people who are smarter than you. We'll be taking a look at the following six signs that will help you determine whether or not that person is smarter than you. One caveat though: they may exhibit one sign and be completely dumb. So, it's important to look for at least two or three signs before making a confirmation.

Here's what you should look for:

They talk less, listen more: This seems like a no brainer thing to do. Most people got smart just by listening to people and speaking at the right opportunities. They can ask questions to gain more information or seek clarification on a statement they're trying to understand.

They specialize in something: A smart person is usually a specialist in one area. Sure, they have interests in broad topics. But there's always that one thing they will talk about for twenty minutes straight and never get tired of doing. They know the ins and outs. They know things about their specialty that most people don't.

Excellent management skills: When a smart person is a leader or a manager, they don't want to be the only smart person in the group. They want their subordinates to gain knowledge and will waste no time spreading that wealth of knowledge with other people. As long as they find people who are willing to learn, it might seem simple enough to do.

Pressing on when things go south: This goes without saying. But smart people are usually disciplined and mentally tough. One such example that proves this is their ability to handle things that don't go in their favor with as little stress as possible. They laugh off simple mistakes and move on instead of dwelling on them. Also, when things go wrong, they always have a few alternative plans up their sleeves. They're like magicians in a sense. What the conflict sees, they are being fooled by the smart person who has already "escaped" with an alternative solution.

They use social media, but not in the usual way: At some point, a smart person will rely on social media as a source of information. They won't engage in any of the petty, toxic stuff that most people will use social media for. They might be on social media for the purpose of communicating with family and close friends. Other than that, a smart person doesn't care much for it.

They don't make people look stupid: A smart person will never make someone look stupid. It would be easy to do, yet there's a caveat. If they try to make a person look bad, that will boomerang back to them and they themselves will look bad as well. Talk about a counterintuitive task. Instead, they try to make them into a smart person.

Now that you know these signs, you will have a less difficult time trying to spot the smartest people you can find. You can come across them by complete accident just by having random conversations with them. Also, getting connected with smart people and building a network will take time and effort. But it will be nice to have on hand knowing you have a question to ask or need to seek some kind of advice.

In this day in age, you can follow people who are smarter than you on social media. Find out what they are reading or sharing. Find ways to connect with them. If they fit your ideal profile of who you want to connect with, then add them to a list of people who you want to meet. These don't have to be big name people at first. If you shoot for the big-name people first, it will be very difficult to connect with them since there are plenty of gatekeepers (not to mention, their busy schedules will be a pain to navigate).

TIPS ON WHAT SMART PEOPLE DO

If you want to become smart and actually know the part, it's important to know what they do (other than the traits listed above). Here are some things that we suggest:

Read: That's what you're doing now, right? Plus, there are other books that you might want to consider reading as well. So long as they are of interest to you, have at it. One more thing, what topic are you interested in gaining knowledge in? Once you have an idea, start by reading some of the best books (along with some related titles).

Dress the part: This may sound a bit ridiculous. But there's usually a pattern of how smart people dress. Usually they are well-dressed, well-groomed, and take good care of themselves. If you follow people who are smarter than you, observe how they are dressed. This doesn't mean you have to wear a suit and tie all the time. But something that makes you look presentable.

Communicate effectively: What's the difference between someone who rushes while they talk and someone who talks slowly, articulately, and pauses at the right moments? One of them is an effective communicator. The person who talks like they are in a hurry don't communicate effectively. And they will often stumble all over the place. Someone who talks slow, gets to the point, and pauses to gather their thoughts before continuing will be perceived as much smarter.

Learn to easily build rapport: When connecting with people who you want to include in your network, building rapport is key. Get to know them a bit. Try not to reach for anything too personal early on in the interaction.

There are plenty of things smart people can do (and so will you with practice). Smart people do things a certain way subconsciously. They weren't born to communicate effectively or have an easy time to build rapport. They've learned it. Smart people know how to build themselves into better versions of themselves.

TAKE THE PROACTIVE APPROACH

A disciplined and smart person is always looking for the proactive approach instead of the reactive. When you are proactive, you are taking responsibility. Those who are proactive don't place blame on other people or things that are within control. Sounds familiar, doesn't it? Reactive people do the exact opposite of what we've just mentioned. Show us someone who is disciplined and reactive and we'll show you someone that has never told a lie in their lifetime.

So, what is the difference between being proactive and reactive? Let's take a look at the following scenario: For example, if some kid called you stupid for no apparent reason, what would you do? A reactive person would justify that they are not stupid and maybe even hassle the kid. A proactive person meanwhile will have that choice to react that way or ignore it and move on. In their heads, they don't care about some bratty kid's opinion. They will usually do the same thing if someone who is an adult called someone stupid for no reason.

The one true difference between a proactive and a reactive person is choice. A reactive person has already chosen to react while a proactive person has a different avenue to travel. It seems like a simple thing to do, but many people don't know nor practice this.

Reactive people will let things that are beyond their control get to them. A proactive person will understand that these exist and there is nothing that they can do. But they know of some alternatives and workarounds. For example, if you're a mom or dad who is planning on taking your son out for a picnic at the park and it rains, you can take him to lunch at your favorite restaurant instead. No big deal, there's always an alternative.

A reactive person will feel bad about not being able to do something with their kids and will feel like they've failed as a parent (when in reality, it's not their fault). Things beyond your control will either influence your behavior or allow you to act accordingly based on alternative plans that you might have laid out in advance (or thought of on the spot).

RECAP

When it comes to discipline, it should be treated as if it were your own child. You want to birth it and nurture it. The last thing you want to do is harm it by making mistakes that seem like harmless tasks (like procrastination). Another thing you shouldn't worry about is finding motivation. Forget the fact that such a thing exists. Just do the task anyways even if you don't feel like doing it. You'll have a sense of accomplishment and know that having a crappy day isn't going to stop you from completing the day's tasks.

Someone who lives a disciplined life possesses traits that can be easily acquired. They are committed to sticking to their goals, placing their emotions in the back seat, and keeping their eye on the prize no matter what. They will do their best to conquer their goals and get the job done no matter what life throws at them.

If you want to learn more about living a more disciplined life, it's best to go to the source: the smartest people you know. They are usually more disciplined and mentally tougher than most. Do your best to connect with them be it online or in person. These will be people you can learn from or even form lifelong friendships with.

Finally, taking the proactive approach instead of a reactive approach will definitely be a boost for your discipline and mental toughness. It will challenge you to handle things beyond your control in a more appropriate manner. You'll learn how to come up with alternative plans when things don't go your way. And you'll learn that it's pointless to blame other people or things on the negative things affecting your life.

A proactive person is smart, sees some good in the bad, and will always come out on top in the end. It's a matter of how they choose to react in a negative situation.

REACHING FOR YOUR HIGHEST GOALS AND AIMING FOR TRUE FREEDOM

E veryone has a goal that is the highest of them all. And for most, achieving it may seem next to impossible. However, as long as they have the right mindset, they can achieve it. In this chapter, we'll be talking about setting those goals, attaining them, and being able to live a life of true freedom.

We'll talk about the things that might move you in the right direction? What will be enough for you to get started and stay in a forward direction. Before you know it, you'll be able to move in the right direction without having any problems. Even with slight setbacks, you'll know exactly what to do and where to go.

This chapter will show you exactly what it takes to reach your goals. You'll learn that there are many ways to set goals and attain them. But for the sake of simplicity, we'll show you one way to approach them with ease. If you want to achieve your goals and easily do so without procrastination, keep reading.

WHAT MOVES YOU?

What is something that moves you? What gets you out of bed in the morning? These are just a couple of questions worth asking. There's always something that you love doing to a point where you get never tired of it. It's the one thing that will turn you from being lazy to a person of action.

Another thing that can move you is influence. However, there are three types of influence that exist: negative, neutral, and positive. Let's face it: influence and control are something we want in our lives. And that's one of the few reasons why you're reading this book right now. You want total control over most things in your life. You want to be free from the entities that tie you down and limit what control you have at the moment.

We also want to set an example for those who seek our influence. The last thing we want to be are bad influences on others. Speaking of seeking influence, you're more likely looking for it yourself. The only kind of influence you want to see are those who are on the positive side. Needless to say, there are positive influences that are watching your every move (and you might not even know it). Who exactly are these positive influences? Your parents, your spouse, your children, anyone who plays a positive and important role in your life.

Naturally, these are the people who will be your best friends and cheerleaders. If you are a parent, your children are watching you. If anything, you are responsible for being the influential figure in their life. So, it would be best for you to set the best example for them possible, so they learn from you.

Whether you know it or not, your actions no matter how big or small will play an influential role. You can influence someone in your life without saying a word. Avoid bad influences as much as you can. Their actions (or inactions) might just draw you in and you may mimic what they're doing. This is something you don't want to do when your ultimate goal is to be your most disciplined and be mentally tough.

WHO ARE YOUR LIFE-CHANGING INFLUENCERS?

Jesus Christ. Mother Teresa. Abraham Lincoln. Elon Musk.

These are just a few names of people that may earn the title of life changing influencers. These historical figures and big names may have a set of words and actions that can impact people in such a positive way. But do your life-changing influencers have to be famous people? Absolutely not. They can be members of your family you have never met in your life.

The truth is, there are a couple people you'll come across in your life who will who will change your life for the better. You will be fortunate to learn from them, admire them, and talk highly about them long after they pass away. Who knows? You could be that life-changing influencer in someone's life. You could be living or dead and still make some kind of impact on a person.

Take a moment to think about your ideal life-changing influencers. Who do you aspire to be more like? What is it about them that draws you to them? Why do you consider them influencers? These are just a few questions that you should consider asking yourself.

There's bound to be one in your life even at this point in your life. Who was one of your favorite teachers in school? Do you consider them to be a disciplined and mentally tough individual? What was it about their classes that drew you to take them? Remember, there is plenty of room for you to include another influencer in your life that will change you for the better.

MOVING AS IF EVERYTHING IS EFFORTLESS

Do you ever watch shows like "American Ninja Warrior" or "Titan"? These are TV shows where people with insane athletic abilities showcase their talents by going through obstacle courses in a timely manner. These are not your usual obstacle courses like running around cones or alternating between feet on a tire course.

These competitors cross through rickety bridges, rappel up walls, and walk through balance beams quickly. If you fall into the mud or water, you lose. To the average person, it seems like a very difficult task to do. But for the contestants of these shows, they have put in plenty of work to make sure they are in top physical condition.

When practicing for these competitions, they practice without making any kind of effort. They also perform tasks that may sound impossible for the average person to do (as if it were almost uncharacteristic of them). They train hard, change their diets to accommodate said training, and put in the work even on days when they don't want to. On top of that, they make sacrifices in order to focus more on their training. The lesson here is they had a system in place where they were able to achieve their goals. Their ultimate goal was to compete in "American Ninja Warrior" or "Titan".

They know that winning it all would be the cherry on top. But just being on there is just enough for them. After all that hard work and dedication, they've made it.

Getting to the point: the lesson is that they have put in the practice and the work to make everything effortless. They are aware of the mistakes they make and how many times they will happen. They don't complain or think that they suck at what they do. They get back up, plow through it, and get it done.

What causes effortless achievement to be "impossible"?

For most of us, our desire to get moving without little to no motivation is what we look for. How great would it be for us to get out of bed in the morning and do something without effort or fail? Unfortunately, that seems to be within a much farther reach. It seems like whenever we want to do something, we don't feel like it and would rather be lazy all day.

Achieving our goals with little to no effort is possible. But how do we get there? The key to go from wanting to do something to doing it anyway can be summed up into these words: emotional understanding. How do you approach emotional understanding?

How this works is you take a look at the goal you want to achieve. From there, you will be able to examine why it's so difficult to achieve it. What makes it so unpleasant? Once you have a good idea of why it seems like such a monumental task to achieve, only then you can disconnect the negative associations from it. Specifically, the negative emotions and associations of doing a goal are usually the "I don't want to do it" or "I don't feel like doing it". Some will even use the excuse of the work being "too hard". That's a sign of emotional resistance. And that's just another sign of letting your emotions control you instead of the other way around.

What you need to do is learn what your emotional blockers are? If your goal is to climb Denali in Alaska, but you're afraid of heights then your fear of heights is an emotional blocker. There are three types of emotional blockers that exist:

Immediate: This kind of emotional blocker stems from what you actually dislike about achieving the goal itself. In other words, what is it about the goal you want to achieve that you hate? Is it something you hate having to do? You need to perform the task anyways no matter how much you're going to hate it. A real-life example of this is not being able to spend time with your family because of an important deadline coming up. While you are not ignoring them in the slightest, you need a lot of time and attention to accomplish a goal that will mean big things for your business. You hate having to sacrifice that time that would otherwise be spent on those you love. But without that sacrifice, you and your family won't be better off.

Identity: This comes down to negative self-talk. "You can't get it done because you're terrible at X." You say to yourself that you're not the type of person to achieve a goal you plan on setting. You can be your own self. But you can be a better version if you achieve the goals you set, even if it's uncharacteristic of you. There's nothing more satisfying than someone telling you that there is something different about you (and in a good way).

Receiving: These are basically certain beliefs that you adopt that are preventing you from the goal you want to achieve. For example, someone may be struggling to achieve a certain task but have too much pride to ask for help. They don't want to be perceived as weak. We're all human. And when humans struggle, they are not afraid to ask for help.

You should take a moment and think about the kind of emotional blockers you have dealt with in the past. It doesn't have to be too long of a list. Think of five different emotional blockers you have dealt with in the past. Think of the goals you want to accomplish and look ahead. What kind of immediate blockers do you see? What are you willing to sacrifice for the sake of reaching your goal (but would find hard to give up)?

What kind of negative self-talk have you given yourself? And lastly, what are the emotional blockers that happen as you move closer to achieving your goal? Are you too proud to ask for help? Are you saying to yourself that such a goal is impossible?

Being able to assess what your emotional blockers are and being able to conquer them will help you become more able to attain your goals without the effort and motivation needed.

ADDITIONAL TIPS FOR EFFORTLESSLY ACHIEVING YOUR GOALS

As you venture towards your journey in achieving your highest goals, you'll want to take the following seven tips below. It's understandable that there are things you don't want to do. At the same time, your negative emotions are mostly to blame for your inaction or slow moving towards the goals you set.

Here are some things to take into consideration:

Delegate it, if need be: Don't know how to do a certain task? Do you know how but don't have the time? Delegate it to someone who will get it done for you. We can't juggle everything all at once. As humans, we have our limits. There are times when a goal that needs to be achieved where it will take more than one person to accomplish it. Delegate to someone who has the skill and competence and you'll feel a lot better.

Eliminate the old goals: You probably have a to do list that has goals that you have never gotten around to or tried to achieve (but never materialized). The only thing to do at this point is eliminate them all together. What's the point in trying to get them done when it's going to sit there and collect dust? Instead, focus on goals that interest you and make you happy.

Know your boundaries: In the previous chapter, we've talked about setting boundaries. It's important to remind yourself what they are and what you need to do to stay within them.

Eliminate distractions: We've already covered distractions earlier on in the book. By now, you should have a basic idea on how to eliminate both external and internal distractions. If not, refer to Chapter 3 on how you can minimize them to your advantage.

Find the right tools for the job: Depending on the goals you want to achieve, it's important to find the right tools that will work. If you are using something that is not working effectively then it would be time to find something that is new, much more functional, and able to get the job done.

Change what isn't working: If you are doing something that isn't working, what's the point in doing the same thing over and over again expecting a different result (which is insanity, of course). Change it up and see if it works. If it does, good. If not, repeat the process until something is working.

Double down on what's working: If you know what is working in terms of achieving your goals, this is a good opportunity to double down on it. If you are putting in the work, you can put in double the work if you are up to the challenge. The more you double down, the faster you can achieve your highest goal without half-assing it or reducing the quality of it.

3 IS A MANAGEABLE NUMBER TO START WORKING ON

Whoever coined the term "it's easy as 1, 2, 3" obviously hit the nail on the head. When you start setting goals that you want to achieve, you want the process to be as simple as possible. Step one, step two, step three, done. Sounds kind of nice, right? In this brief section, we'll show you a three-step newbie-friendly way to set the goals you want to achieve. Later on in the chapter, we'll talk about the different methods of goal setting that you can use.

Now, here is the three-step process to help you set your goals so you can achieve them with ease:

1. **Set three manageable goals:** Seems simple enough, right? Three simple goals that you can easily attain in a short amount of time would be a good start. Five goals would be pushing it. Ten might be torture (especially if you are starting out).
2. **Make sure they are high, but attainable:** You want the goals to be a bit of a challenge. But nothing too difficult. You want them to stretch a bit. If you don't, they will likely be considered "to-do" items and not goals.
3. **Put together a series of "To-Dos" in one list:** You can set "to-do" tasks into a list that can form that goal you want to achieve. The best technique for something like this is the SMART technique (which we will learn in the next section).

THERE ARE MULTIPLE WAYS TO SET YOUR GOALS, BUT YOU SHOULD CHOOSE ONE THAT WORKS BEST FOR YOU

In this section, we'll be talking about three goal management methods that will work to your advantage. They include the following:

SMART, HARD, and WOOP. You're probably wondering "what the heck are they"? We'll break down each method so you have a better understanding of what they are and how you can use them. First, let's break down SMART:

THE SMART METHOD

Wasting no time, let's take a look at SMART:

Specific: What is the specific goal that you want to achieve? Rather than be vague about it like say "make more money" you can say "Make $10,000 by December 31st by starting a content marketing agency for eCommerce stores". Or instead of "lose weight", you can say you want to "lose 10 pounds in six weeks by working out three times a week for 15 minutes". The more specific you whittle it down to, the better.

Measurable: You obviously need to keep track of your goals. And one of the best ways to do it is measure them. You won't be able to know how far you've gotten if you don't have the metrics or the data. Without them, you won't be able to determine whether or not making a change towards achieving your goal is possible.

Attainable: If your goal is realistic, it can be attainable. How long can you achieve the goal itself? Don't set lofty goals and think you can achieve it in the quickest amount of time possible. If you want to earn $10,000 (for example), think of a realistic time frame. Can you do it in six months? Possible, but it will be difficult. How about a year? Sounds realistic enough.

Relevant: Is this goal relative to your values? Is this the kind of goal that will make you happy? Does it fall in line with your personal beliefs? These are some of the questions you need to ask yourself to ensure that your goals are relevant to you.

Time-bound: It's always a good idea to set a timeframe to when the goal can be achieved. You can't say you want to do X and Y without a specific time frame. Again, think realistically here. For smaller goals, set a shorter time frame. For example, if you want to lose five pounds, six weeks might be a good time frame. If you want to lose 20 pounds, consider three months might be good enough.

THE HARD TECHNIQUE

Next, we'll be taking a look at the HARD technique. Here's what HARD stands for:

Heartfelt: Sometimes, investing your emotions towards your goals may be necessary. Why do you care about this goal? What is your emotional attachment? Is it because of someone you love? What's that one emotion that's driving you to achieve that goal?

Animated: This will help you think ahead to what will occur after the fact. Visualize yourself in a scene where you have just achieved the goal of your dreams. How do you feel? What kind of emotions are you sensing?

Required: What are the concrete reasons that are helping you achieve those goals? What has to get done? What goals need to be done urgently?

Difficulty: This is where you really want to challenge yourself. You intentionally want to make the goal difficult so you can face the challenges head on. Although, we stress that you shouldn't make it harder than it has to be. Set some challenges that can be difficult to accomplish. But be aware of the challenge ahead so you can prepare yourself to conquer it at every opportunity.

THE WOOP TECHNIQUE

Lastly, we'll take a look at the WOOP Technique: This is perfect for when you want to break old habits and form new ones. Let's get right to it:

Wish: What goal are you excited about achieving? What is it that you dream about? Think of what it is and be sure that it is a realistic enough goal to achieve.

Outcome: What is the outcome that you want to achieve? Picture it in your mind.

Obstacle: What obstacles will stand in the way of this goal? Being aware of them before you even move forward will put you at a greater advantage of going up against them. You can navigate the obstacles with ease and simplicity. You'll know about what could hold you back. At the same time, you'll need to form a battle plan to attack the obstacles and move forward.

Plan: Without a plan, you do nothing. Plan the initial steps you need to take. Plan some alternatives in case you hit some dead-ends or obstacles. Planning ahead of time will put you at an even greater advantage.

One of these techniques can work to your advantage. It's important to test one out and see which one will be more effective. As mentioned before, the WOOP technique is perfect for anyone looking to form a new habit while kicking old ones to the curb. If you are looking to start a new online business and plan on growing it over time, the SMART technique might be better suited for such a thing.

DEFINE YOUR FREEDOM AND BE ACCOUNTABLE

True freedom is worth accomplishing. You want to break free from the prison that is your mind of a negative mindset. The late Sean Stephenson once said that your mind is like a prison. You can escape it at any time since there is no guard or barb wire fence. But what keeps you inside that prison is your limiting self-belief.

The truth is, you can acquire true freedom just by busting out of that prison. From there, you are free to move in any direction. So long as it takes you to your ultimate destination (your main goal). Freedom is possible, but the only obstacle standing in our way is ourselves.

Freedom is different from one person to the other. One person wants to be free in spirit. The other wants to attain freedom in the sense of not being tied down by their financial issues. Freedom is not some kind of political term. It's something that can be acquired in a physical, spiritual, and psychological sense. You can physically free yourself from a life of potential health issues by losing weight. You can be free from psychological setbacks and mental blocks if you decide to push forward and change your mindset for the better.

The one thing you need to know about acquiring freedom is having awareness. You must be aware that you aren't completely free until you've taken the steps to achieve it. Once you are aware of your newfound freedom, the mission is accomplished. Awareness is the first and last step.

In this instance, you are aware that you are not in the right mindset. You are not in a state where you are disciplined or mentally tough to handle life's challenges. Prison is hell (literally and figuratively). In this context, living a life where discipline and mental toughness does not exist might be your own personal hell. You can break free from comfort and complacency. You can escape negativity with the right kind of escape plan that is being outlined in this book.

Jocko Wilinik said it best: discipline equals freedom. To translate it in plain English, as long as you have control you will have freedom. Control over your mindset, your daily habits, and everything in between. If you accept discipline, you earn freedom. Jocko is disciplined enough to get up every morning at 4:30 AM, allowing him more time in the day. You don't have to get up early in the morning to attain this.

If you want financial freedom, you must instill financial discipline. Stop spending your money on needless things. You can save money and have it ready in a moment's notice when some not so pleasant financial situation rears its ugly head. You will have the freedom to get rid of it quickly before the problem gets worse. Holding yourself accountable and making sure that you make intelligent financial decisions will ensure that you keep up with your usual expenses, so you don't find yourself in a jeopardizing situation (such as eviction from your home).

HOW TO HOLD YOURSELF ACCOUNTABLE

Holding yourself accountable is one of the key skills to have in order to achieve true freedom. Failure to do so will lessen your chances. Here are some tips that you should follow in order to hold yourself more accountable now and in the future:

Don't reveal your goals: One of the most fatal mistakes anyone can make is revealing their goals and intentions to anyone. The more they disclose, the more pressure you'll put on yourself (especially when people ask you how things are going). Remember, you never know who is watching you actually attain that specific goal you set forth. Contrary to popular belief, announcing your goals is not the best way to hold yourself accountable. People want premature praise for an accomplishment that may never materialize. Not only that, you may receive negative feedback before you even move forward with your goal. And that alone could mentally paralyze someone and thus they never start in the first place.

Write down your goals: If you have a goal that you want to achieve, put it to paper. Better yet, start with a major goal and put together a simple list on how you want to achieve it. These include your short-term and long-term goals. Make sure you have it written nice and neat on a piece of paper or notebook.

Put together a mission statement: A mission statement defines who you are, the goals you want to achieve, and the values you hold dear. No need for it to be long like a novel. Keep it short, sweet, and to the point.

Review your overall performance: Taking a look at how you performed overall will give you a view at what you've done right, what you've done wrong, and what you can do to improve at the next opportunity.

Don't be afraid to ask for feedback: Feedback is important. Ask your fellow team members or your support network. You will get positive feedback. But not all of it will be positive at all. Use the negative feedback as an opportunity to make some changes and adjustments where necessary.

SELF-DISCIPLINE CAN CREATE MORE FREEDOM THAN EVER BEFORE IN YOUR LIFE

This can't be stressed enough. Being able to discipline yourself will help you create the kind of freedom that you want. Self-discipline allows you to gain control and therefore gives you the freedom to do whatever you want. Freedom allows you flexibility, indulgence, and allowance. So, the two go hand in hand.

Simply put, discipline is the giver of freedom. It is never a taker. That is why it is important to put yourself first to an extent. But in some situations, putting yourself last is equally as important. If you are a parent, you always put your family first. It's all about making the right decision that will benefit not just you but the most important people in your life.

Self-discipline will force you to make decisions that may be hard, but in the end, they were good decisions. For example, if you are trying to live a healthy lifestyle, it may seem tough to give up the fast food. But instead of going for that number one with a Coke, you opt for a salad and a bottle of water instead. It's hard to let go of the things you are used to. But in the end, it's worth it. Learn to embrace these kinds of decisions and you'll make them without breaking a sweat.

The question for you is simply this: how far are you willing to go to attain self-discipline? What are you willing to give up? What are you most passionate about focusing on? The reward of freedom is sweet when you are consistent with self-discipline.

INDULGE IN YOUR GREATEST PLEASURE AND HOBBIES 'GUILT FREE' AND WITHOUT ANY FORM OF PROCRASTINATION

When you are self-disciplined, you will be able to do more instead of less. You will get to enjoy doing the things that you love. The goals that you want to achieve are easy to attain. You can be able to work on that passion project that you've been putting off for so long. You will feel no shame. And you will not feel the need to procrastinate.

It's important to let in what you want to bring into your life and let out what you want to get rid of. It's hard to let go of the things you've once enjoyed. But once you realize it was more of a waste of time than a true return on investment, you'll realize that letting it go won't be so bad after all.

RECAP

Being able to reach for your highest goals and attaining true freedom in the process is possible. It all boils down to being disciplined enough to get it done. As someone who is on the path towards discipline and mental toughness, you realize that you are setting an example for those keeping a close eye on you. You will develop into a positive influence for someone important in your life. Plus, you also model yourself after the people in your life who are considered life changing influencers.

Being able to move towards your goal without a lot of effort will come down to one thing: being able to be consistent and put in the work. Don't worry about making mistakes or the setbacks that happen. As long as you are aware of those setbacks, you'll be ready for them whether they pop up or not. Think of yourself as someone who is competing for American Ninja Warrior. Your goal that you want to attain is at the other end of the course.

When managing your goals, it's as easy as 1,2,3 in planning them. However, you'll want to consider a method to set your goals. Whether you want to be SMART about it or WOOP it up, there's a method that will work for just about anyone.

Your freedom is your reward for being self-disciplined and holding yourself accountable. This will allow you to give yourself more time to work on a passion project, more financial freedom and the ability to knock out any financial problems before they worsen, and the freedom to do whatever you feel like doing. The freedom to do something is possible to attain so long as you are willing to discipline yourself.

IV

LEARN TO LOVE THE PROCESS, YOU CAN'T SKIP IT

DEVELOPING DISCIPLINE

This chapter will cover step by step on how you should develop discipline. If anything, it should be built block by block. It should be like a brick wall or a tall building. The higher it goes, the higher your level of discipline is. Discipline will help you focus on the tasks that you want to get done while allowing you to develop the ability to restrain yourself from veering off course.

We'll talk about whether or not motivation is enough or not. We'll also talk about what discipline should not be used for. The power of discipline is useful in many situations. But there are times when it may not be needed. We'll also talk about how to handle your urges and how you should simply "ride the wave" instead of being swallowed by it.

This chapter will show you how to make the easy and hard choices without breaking a sweat. The decision making we face on a regular basis can be as simple as ordering a pizza or as difficult as crossing a high wire. Even making the toughest decisions possible may seem effortless (even in situations where either decision will yield some kind of negative consequence).

Lastly, you will learn the kind of self-discipline developed by professional athletes and Navy SEALs. These are the type of people who face monumental tasks on a regular basis. And they do the hard things without fail or little effort needed. This chapter is something you really want to pay attention to. Especially when you want to develop discipline. Let's begin:

MOTIVATION IS GOOD AND ALL, BUT IT IS NOT ENOUGH

Early in the book, we stated that motivation is something that is elusive if you search for it. We also said that you don't need to find motivation to start on a task. Do it anyways even if you don't feel like it. Motivation is like a cat. It comes to you at times when you least expect it.

Even if motivation finds you, it won't be enough. However, there are some links to the chain that you want to add. We'll be talking about aspiration and dedication. Both of these are what you need aside from motivation itself to achieve the tasks that are set forth. Putting the three together will mix into the perfect blend of discipline.

Let's discuss each of these things starting with aspiration:

The Importance of Aspiration

Aspiration is defined as the ambition or hope of achieving a specific goal or task. In a team setting, the goals and targets that you as a team set forth can be accomplished with ease if they are aligned within your aspirations. When that happens, the engagement levels will increase. The team will work together as one giant unit.

Before the team works together, they need to know what's in it for them. What exactly will be the end goal for the team? How will they be rewarded for a job well done? If there is nothing they get in return, what's the point in working together?

When a team knows that there is a reward at the end of the tunnel, the team will work together. So long as there are no personal differences that will affect the team's morale or the like, the team can accomplish the goal in front of them. One of our basic needs that need to be met according to the Maslow Hierarchy is the sense of achievement and recognition for what we do. It doesn't matter if you work as part of a team or achieve something in terms of individual efforts. There is no better feeling like accomplishing something of value and being recognized for it. The problem is most people decide to let it go unnoticed.

Aspiration is one of the key things that you need in order to be disciplined. What is your biggest aspiration? How will you achieve it? What obstacles will likely stand in the way of it? And what will you do to conquer those obstacles and move forward?

Why is dedication equally important?

Dedication and motivation are not the same. Dedication is making a decision and honoring it at every possible opportunity. You are committed to starting the goal or task and seeing it through to the end. It is dedication that separates those who are the true winners from those who just quit when things go south.

Dedication is what happens when motivation is nowhere to be found, but you do the work anyways. Because the sooner you complete a task or get closer to your goal, the better you'll feel knowing you've made the right decision. When things go wrong, you don't give up. When you fall off the horse, you get back up and ride again. That is what dedication is all about.

When you or your team is faced with setbacks, it's important to assess what they are and handle them accordingly. After that, you keep pressing forward. You don't stop, drop everything, and call it good. When the job is half done, it's not good enough. There will be those on the team that may quit on you halfway through. Either you carry on and let someone take on a bit of an extra load. Or find someone who is competent and positive enough to take on the challenges that still lie ahead for the team.

Dedication is one thing that no living individual can ever ignore or exclude from recognizing someone's achievements.

DISCIPLINE SHOULD NOT BE USED FOR ACTIVITIES & TASKS LIKE THIS…

One of the things where discipline should not be used is when you are doing creative activities. Creativity is more of a process instead of a discipline. Discipline teaches you to keep within your boundaries and limits. With creativity, there are a set of rules that can be followed. However, you can break them as you please. They mostly won't care for limitations and will likely branch off on different paths in search of new discoveries. You often see this with artists and musicians. They hate being able to keep within the normal boundaries and rules. So, they dare to walk a tight line and create something that takes things a step further.

You can use discipline when doing creative things. But at the same time, you don't have to be a follower of any rules. It sounds like a paradox because discipline and rules seem to go hand in hand. Discipline and creativity shall never meet. Any creative project will seem like a job if you incorporate discipline. Creativity in one aspect is like discipline: it gives you freedom. In this context, you have the freedom to let your creativity run wild. When the inspiration hits you, you add something to what you're currently creating or start from scratch. Either way, the rules won't apply, and discipline is not necessary in this regard.

RIDING THE WAVE OF YOUR URGES

In this section, we're going to talk about "urge surfing". What is it exactly? It's basically addressing impulsive behaviors. Specifically, they are mostly associated with addictions such as binge eating or drinking large amounts of alcohol on a regular basis. When you feel the need to have a drink or eat a lot to deal with a negative emotion, it's easy just to give in and get it done.

But with urge surfing, it's an entirely different thing. This is a mindfulness technique that you can use to your advantage each time you have an urge. You don't act on that addictive behavior. Instead, you meditate and let it pass through you. This is a lot better than trying to fight it.

How do you do this mindfulness technique? First off, close your eyes. Imagine that you are riding on a surfboard. That giant wave you are riding is your urge. Imagine riding the ups and downs of that wave. You are closing in on the shoreline that will guide you towards freedom and discipline. Typically, an urge will last 20 to 30 minutes.

Any pro surfer can tell you that you can ride the wave with ease, or you can make one wrong move and the wave comes crashing down on you. With urge surfing, whatever you don't do will get weaker (and whatever you do will get stronger). The more you act on your urge, the stronger it gets (and vice versa).

Urge surfing for best results

This urge surfing technique will allow you to meditate for intervals of one to five minutes. After each interval, you should reassess your urge. If you are still feeling it, repeat the process. You'll start to notice that urge subsiding little by little as you go. Doing this repeatedly will help you break that connection between you and the urge itself.

Alternatives to consider

Even though riding the urge wave is one thing to handle it, you should also consider other alternatives in order for it to pass. For example, you can talk to a friend or family member for a while. Or you can watch something educational on YouTube. Do something that will help you get your mind off of the urge and focused on something else.

The easier you are able to do this, the better you'll be able to handle any urge no matter how sudden it appears. You can perform these tasks in between meditation sessions if you wish. From time to time, you should check to see if the urge is still existent.

Urge surfing is the perfect way for you to gain control over your urges. You can literally suck the power right out of your urges and beat them into submission with ease once you get the hang of it.

MAKING YOUR CHOICE, EITHER IT'S EASY OR HARD

We face countless decisions every single day. Most of them are usually easy. Some of them may be hard. But in the end, it's you that determines whether or not that decision is either or. You can make it easy on yourself or harder than it has to be. It's true that there are some decisions you make that will be tough because of the ramifications that follow. For example, a manager may be faced with the task of letting go of one employee due to cutbacks. The company is hemorrhaging money, and someone may need to be let go just to save money.

Sometimes, the hard decisions can yield some positive results no matter how unpopular it is in the eyes of other people. In terms of growth and discipline, making the decisions you hate is a likely thing to happen.

HOW TO MAKE BETTER DECISIONS

Having the ability to make better decisions even under pressure will put you at a greater advantage compared to others. We'll be taking a look at the following tips below, so you'll be able to make better decisions. Even high-pressure decisions can be made with little effort as possible. Let's take a look at these tips:

1. **Always go with your gut:** This should be rule number one in anyone's decision making rule book. You'd be crazy to go against your gut. It will never steer you wrong 99 percent of the time. Your gut will be able to tell you what's right and what's wrong before your consciousness even gets to it. Unconscious decision making can save your hide in the most high-pressure situations. If you get that "funny" feeling when faced with a potential life-altering decision, then you'll want to address it. Don't even dare to ignore it.

2. **You don't always have to ask everyone:** It's admirable to ask people for their opinion on something before making a decision. However, if it's a high-pressure decision you'll face more problems when you hear two different opinions. One person tells you to do it and the other tells you not to. And that's where the pressure gets cranked up to another

level. Sometimes, it's better to never seek the opinion of others at all.

3. **Ask yourself the right questions:** How will this decision benefit me and the others? What will be the outcome if I make decision A? What about decision B? These are questions you'll want to ask yourself. It's good to carefully weigh the pros and cons of each decision. Sometimes, either decision is a lose-lose. It's a matter of what kind of repercussions will deal a lesser blow once the decision itself is made.

4. **Consider your values:** It's easy to make a decision so long as it aligns with your values. However, there may be decisions where neither of them will be on par with them. It's important to know what your core values are and how they define your life. Write down a list of your highest values. Make sure that it is clear and easy to understand. That way, whenever you need to fall back on them for references, you'll have a good idea of what you believe in. Especially when it comes to making the right kind of decisions.

5. **Be aware of the effects:** Each decision has an effect that will alter the course of future events. Imagine that you're about to give a presentation to investors for the purpose of getting more capital for your business. But there is one problem: you have a fear of public speaking. If you back out now because of your fears, you'll never get the capital you need, and your business will suffer. Press on and get through it, you can impress them enough to get the money. Even if

the investors say no, at least you faced your fear. And you understood that impact of making the right decision even if it means doing something you're afraid of. Because there is something greater than your fear. In this instance, it was a brighter financial future for you personally and for your business.

6. **Visualize the future with every decision:** We cannot stress visualization enough. It's important to imagine in your head the scene that can unfold with each decision you make. Try to tie in the emotion of it while you're at it. This will help you make a decision that may be a painful one. Also, if you feel that a certain decision doesn't feel so bad compared to the other, that's when you know that it could be the right one even if the outcome is rather sucky for you and the others.

7. **Get both sides of your brain involved:** Emotions and logic should come into account here. Engaging one side of your brain won't be enough. The goal here is to find a balance of emotion and reason with the decisions you make.

SECRETS USED BY NAVY SEALS & PROFESSIONAL ATHLETES TO DEVELOP UNBEATABLE SELF DISCIPLINE THAT MAKES DOING "HARD" TASKS INCREDIBLY EFFORTLESS

The US Navy SEALs are one of the most dangerous fighting forces in the known world. They have traveled the world over and taken part in missions where every decision they make was hard and complex.

Yet, they seem to make it look effortless by deciding the best course of action and acting on it. Professional athletes have a similar mindset that helps them make tough decisions look effortless. When the game is on the line and you're faced with a high-pressure situation, you need to be ready to make snap decisions that can result in winning the game or losing it.

You need to discipline yourself and resist the urge to crack under pressure or give up. You'll want to free yourself from the inability to press on. To quote what Jocko Wilinik said earlier, "discipline equals freedom". And Wilinik himself was a Navy SEAL, so he knows this very well.

We'll be taking a look at some of the secrets that both Navy SEALs and professional athletes know about making hard tasks as effortless as possible. Of course, it all boils down to self-discipline. They know things that we don't (until now). Here's what they are:

Start early

They say the early bird gets the worm. Those words can't be spoken with more truth. The task at hand must be done at some point during the day. You can't cut it too close before the deadline. The sooner you get it done, the better. Not to mention, you have more freedom to do what you want for the rest of the day. Starting early will give you more freedom so long as you don't procrastinate and waste time.

Stay in the moment

This is a big one. When you stay in the moment, you'll never lose sight of the prize. Don't look back and never look sideways. You'll get distracted and thrown off course. When you focus and keep it that way, you'll inch closer towards the goal without even caring how much time has elapsed and the like.

Take good care of yourself

Seems simple enough. You need to take care of yourself both mentally and physically. When you do, the two will work together in perfect harmony. When you do something that is physically challenging, your mind may play tricks on you if it's not completely aligned. You won't be able to manage the pain or endure the challenges that take a long time to complete. The key here is to keep pushing without killing yourself or going crazy.

Take care of your body, don't give into the bad habits and vices, and you will certainly give yourself peace of mind in knowing that you can accomplish whatever tasks you set forth. Also, keeping yourself in good shape physically can keep the mind sharp. Don't forget that.

Understand the importance of detail

Navy SEALs are known for their razor-sharp attention to detail. Everything needs to look perfect in its own way. Make your bed with no wrinkles. Anything that's the least bit crooked and you have to do it over again until you get it right. It's important that you focus on the details. Even the tiny ones. This doesn't mean you have to be a perfectionist. But you have to cover as many bases as possible. Nothing needs to be half-done. And subpar quality does not equal good enough.

Focus on one thing at a time

When you are putting in the practice, focus on one thing at a time. For example, if you are practicing for a presentation you can, do one slide at a time. Say what you need to say. Do it repeatedly before moving on. Do the same thing repeatedly over and over again and fine tune it if needed. Don't overload yourself. Focus on one thing and move onto the next. Rinse and repeat.

If you're surrounded by undisciplined people, do the opposite

Look around you. If you see a lot of people around you that are undisciplined, then do the exact opposite. Stand out above the rest of the "Herd". But when you are surrounded by people who are disciplined, that's when you work together. A lot of people decide to be undisciplined. But you don't have to be. Either you swim with the current or against it.

RECAP

Motivation is something that will come to you rather than something you have to find. Even if you have the motivation, it still won't be enough. You'll want to be able to have aspirations and dedication to compliment motivation. These are the building blocks that will create a potent mixture of discipline.

When it comes to your creativity, discipline should not even be part of the equation. Be creative and enjoy a different kind of freedom without submitting to the rules. Being creative is the only time where discipline is not needed.

If you are dealing with urges, it's important to ride the wave of urges instead of getting swallowed whole by it. Use the mindful technique we've outlined in the chapter. While you're at it, consider doing other things that will mentally reroute your thoughts rather than keep it stuck on the urge that you're trying to avoid. Don't fight it, but ride it instead of giving in.

Making decisions that are tough will need to be effortless. Only you can decide whether or not the decision is easy to swallow or harder than it needs to be. Use your instincts, consider the potential ramifications of each decision, and choose one that may have negative effects, but doesn't deliver a devastating blow to one's morale.

The secrets that Navy SEALs and pro athletes use that we've unveiled can be adapted into your life when disciplining yourself. Start early and ahead of the pack. Stay in the moment and keep at it no matter how tough it gets. Take the best care of yourself. Pay close attention to detail and make sure things look good. And always focus on one thing at a time when practicing. Take it slow and don't overload yourself with many things.

Developing discipline takes time. And it takes a good amount of strength and willpower to get through the obstacles that stand in the way. If you learn how to embrace the suck, you will make every "hard thing" a lot easier, even if it's painful to do.

STRENGTHENING MENTAL TOUGHNESS

Now that you have a game plan to build discipline, we'll now focus on how you can strengthen your mental toughness. In this chapter, we will give you the ultimate guide on how you can build it up from start to finish. When it comes to discipline, mental toughness must exist to complement it.

Mental toughness is the same as physical toughness. In this context, it will take time and consistency to build up the strength. The more time you put into the gym, the stronger you become. With mental toughness, you can train yourself to handle the tough, high-pressure situations when others choose not to.

We'll give you some not so secret recipes on how to build mental toughness from the ground up. You'll learn what to include for the key ingredients that will cultivate into developing the strongest most fortified mentality you can put together. You can develop mental toughness, but not without a proven roadmap to get you from point A to point B. This chapter is exactly that.

Let's continue on with your journey:

THE NOT-SO-SECRET RECIPE FOR MENTAL TOUGHNESS

What we'll be taking a look at next is the not so secret recipe for mental toughness. These are the ingredients to living a mentally tough life. So long as you practice some of the following traits listed below, you will be able to maintain mental toughness for the rest of your days. Whether you are 30 or 60 years old, mental toughness lives on forever. Here are some of the ingredients that make up mental toughness:

- 1 complaint-free attitude
- 1-part mindfulness
- 1 full amount of control
- Dozens of self-respect and mindfulness
- 1-part talent
- 1-part ability
- Substitute bad habits with good strong habits
- Replace "yes" with "no"
- Substitute toxic people with your support network.

For best results, mix these ingredients and "slow cook" them for an unspecified amount of time. Don't worry about how long this will take you. The more you "cook" these ingredients together, the better your mental toughness will turn out and will last a long time.

Let's take a look in-depth as to why these ingredients should be included.

DON'T COMPLAIN

Complaining is a reflection of a poor attitude. There's no other way to say it. Especially when you complain about the trivial things. Someone who is mentally weak will often complain about the slightest changes. They will always look for things to complain about instead of finding the positive.

Not to mention, it's usually the things they can't control that they complain most about. The reality is that there is nothing you can do about it since it's way out of your hands.

KNOW THAT YOU HAVE CONTROL

We've said it before, and we'll say it again. The key to living with mental toughness is having control. You have control over your attitude, your fear, what you let in and what you let out. You can be able to control the things that will define you personally. Even if you feel like you're not in control, it's better to act as if you are than never at all.

MINDFULNESS IS KEY

Being mindful is one of the key components of mental toughness. You can take five minutes out of your day to meditate and remind yourself that you are in control of your thoughts. You can silence the noise in your mind when you take control of it. The more mindful you are, the better.

RESPECT YOURSELF

Those who respect themselves are often mentally tougher than those who don't. When you have respect for yourself, your self-talk will reflect that. No living person in the world can talk to themselves negatively and respect themselves at the same time. When it comes to self-talk, they are positive and use the right words subconsciously. Sometimes, they say it repeatedly in the form of affirmations, so it's embedded in their minds.

SELF-CONFIDENCE

Confidence is something that you must have in order to be mentally tough. You cannot seek it from outside sources (i.e. -- someone's opinion of you). To build self-confidence, you expose yourself to situations where you can be able to rise to the challenge, perform the necessary tasks, and complete them. The more "can do" that you have, the more confident you will become. It will put you on the path going from saying "I can't" to "I can".

HARNESSING YOUR EXISTING TALENT

Maybe you have an existing talent that you want to put to good use. And eventually, you want to improve it to keep yourself sharp. When you are mentally tough, you know that you have enough of the talent to perform the appropriate task. But no matter how good you are, usually there's always improvement to do better. Think of it like Windows. It's updated on a regular basis, even if it's something minor like ironing out a few bugs.

KNOW THAT YOU HAVE THE ABILITY

We've already covered about having the "can do" to perform a task. If you know that you have the ability, that gives you a boost in confidence. Even if you don't know how, give yourself the opportunity to learn. When you learn, you develop a skill that you can do on your own time. The more abilities you have, the more you can say "I can do that".

EMBRACING "NO"

Most people tend to view "no" as the devil. When in reality, it can be the most powerful word to say when you want to discipline yourself. Sure, there may be a negative emotion when you say no to the things you enjoy in favor of something that will benefit you in the long run. But in the end, you'll feel like you've made the right decision by saying no. It will become a lot easier to say "no" to things that are not important to you.

BE WILLING TO LEARN FROM YOUR MISTAKES

Everyone makes mistakes. No one is perfect. There is no other way to say it. And anyone who says otherwise is lying to you. But the real question is: how will you handle your mistakes? Those who are mentally tough acknowledge their mistakes, learn from them, and move on. The exact opposite of this is dwelling on them, complaining about them, and developing a fear to take action because they are afraid of making mistakes over and over again. Mistakes happen. Just be prepared to make them, embrace them, and dissect them for the purpose of learning from them.

TAKE RESPONSIBILITY FOR YOUR ACTIONS, WORDS, ETC.

It's mind-boggling to see that a lot of people don't take responsibility for their actions or what they say. They find the easy way out by blaming other people or things that are way beyond their control. These are the signs of mentally weak individuals. But you can be the exact opposite of this. When you screw up, it's important to approach it with the following attitude: "how can I make it better and what can be done so the same mistake isn't made again?"

ELIMINATE THE TOXIC PEOPLE FROM YOUR LIFE

If there is something that will throw you off your game, it's toxic people. They will spew negativity towards you. They could be bad mouthing or mocking someone else (or even you). You don't have time for that. Nor will you allow anyone to bring you down to their level. Cut them out of your life without shame. If it's so-called "friends", they'd be easy to dump. But if it's members of your family that are toxic, distance yourself from them as far as possible.

DESTROY YOUR BAD HABITS

Bad habits control our mentality for the worse. And it's easy for those to allow them to take control of us. You can't destroy your bad habits if you can't take control. Use the WOOP technique that you've learned early on in the book to break the bad habits and replace them with new ones. Develop good strong habits in their place. So long as you stay motivated and maintain consistency with these good habits, you'll do just fine.

FACT: IT IS EASY TO TELL SOMEONE TO BE POSITIVE, BUT DIFFICULT TO APPLY IT ON YOURSELF

For whatever reason, you can tell someone to be positive. However, you can't bring it to yourself to live by your own advice. That's kind of like telling someone to save their money so they can become a millionaire (but in reality, your money situation isn't the best). They tell you to be positive, but they never show you how to do it. This is where a lot of people end up failing. They don't have the road map to acquire that positive mindset.

Of course, you'll find exactly that in this book (and in this exact section as well). What you'll also get out of thinking positive are a lot of benefits both in the mental and physical sense. Those who live a positive life are less likely to develop certain health issues later on in their lifetime.

BE WISE IN DISTRIBUTING ENERGY

Distributing energy on tasks that are important will be essential. Especially when you need to get the tasks you need done. So, you do not want to focus on wasting energy on the activities that don't matter. This is why procrastination is such a momentum killer (not to mention an energy drainer). Sure, it's tempting to play video games or binge watch your favorite shows on Netflix. However, when you've finished the season finale, it would be hard for you to get started on the tasks that you were supposed to finish the day before.

When the day begins, focus on the critical tasks. When they are done, check your to do list to see what else can be done before the due date. Another thing, be sure to delegate any tasks that may not require your energy since you have other things to focus on.

THE TRUTH ABOUT WILLPOWER, AND HOW TO APPLY THIS KNOWLEDGE TO YOUR ADVANTAGE

What you need to know about willpower is that it is something that you will be exercising for much of your journey. Discipline and mental toughness will rely on willpower more often than not. If you can resist the urge to not get distracted, only then will you be able to harness the true willpower that is inside you. Remember, a lot of us have willpower inside of ourselves. But the only difference is that there are two kinds of people: those who are willing to tap into that supply of willpower and those who are not able to do so (because they don't know it yet).

In a later chapter, we will show you a prime example of willpower in what is known as delayed gratification. We'll explain exactly what that is and how it ties into willpower.

HONING YOUR TALENTS AND ABILITIES TO ITS BEST FORM

Your talents and abilities can be upgraded to its best form. The more you practice them to make them even better, the more you will be able to put them to good use when it comes to achieving the tasks you are good at. This will not only reinforce your confidence in doing things flawlessly, but it will ensure that you have the mental toughness to perform your abilities and talents at the highest level. You know that even if there is little room for error, you'll be able to get the job done without fail.

You can improve your skills at the current level you're at right now and be better. You may be happy with your current skill level, but there may always be room for improvement no matter what.

YOUR CONFIDENCE STARTS WITHIN, NOT ON WHAT SOMEBODY ELSE SAYS

When it comes to confidence, no one can produce it better than you. It is unnecessary to rely on external sources. What we mean by this is this: it's a complete waste of time to try and seek approval from other people. Others' opinions of you should not define your level of confidence. Your abilities and talents do. If you can get the job done, you know you can do it again. You have the confidence to perform the same task over and over again and produce great results in the process.

People will speak highly of you and have your opinion of you in a positive light. You can graciously accept that. But if someone criticizes you negatively, you can choose to ignore it or let it dampen your spirits and confidence. It would be smart of you to ignore the naysayers and keep pressing on as if you never heard it.

USE MENTAL TOUGHNESS TO DEVELOP LASTING HEALTHY AND POSITIVE HABITS IN ALL AREAS OF LIFE

Mental toughness is needed when you want to focus on all aspects in your life. Whether it's with physical fitness, your abilities and talents, or being a better friend or family member using mental toughness to better yourself and building good habits will be effective. You can build habits that will not only focus on one area, but it can also be connected to other areas of your life as well. With a healthy lifestyle thanks to positive habits, it can also allow you to live longer and therefore give you more time to spend with your family. That alone will also help you strengthen your bond with those who are important people in your life.

EMBRACING YOUR IMPERFECTIONS

Whether we're born with them or not, imperfections are a blessing in disguise. Some of these imperfections are things that we cannot control. And that's OK. The best that you can do is see the positive in the potential negative. Rather than let imperfections get the best of you, you keep doing your best. Now, people may talk negatively about your imperfections and say that you can't do such things because of them. But it's all talk. And only the mentally tough with imperfections do not allow that negativity to get the best of them.

MORE SECRETS FROM NAVY SEALS & PROFESSIONAL ATHLETES THAT YOU SHOULD PUT INTO USE

As promised, we'll be taking a look at more secrets from Navy SEALs and professional athletes that will help you become more mentally tough. Earlier, we've discussed that discipline equals freedom. The Navy SEALs have a motto that they live by on a daily basis. The motto is "The Easy Day Was Yesterday". Sure enough, each day can be more challenging than the last. For this reason, you can expect the next day to present you with even tougher challenges. Because the next day will be a lot harder compared to the last.

One other secret that we want to share is something that Navy SEALs still use to this day. This is known as the "40 percent rule". The rule states that when you feel tapped out after getting 40 percent of the work done, know that you have 60 percent left in the tank. Even if you are tapped out, you have it within you to finish what you started. There is no quit in you. If you ever think about quitting, don't.

THERE'S A GOOD KIND OF STRESS THAT YOU SHOULD USE

Did you know that there are two kinds of stress out there? There is good stress (eustress) and bad stress (distress). Of course, you need to use the good stress to your advantage. The reason why is that it will give you an energy boost to keep going, even when the pressure is on. Though it is short-term, it will be exactly what you need to speed on through the home stretch. How long does it last? It's anyone's guess. But as long as you use it to get the tasks done, nothing can stop you.

Distress on the other hand will derail you and cause you to crack under pressure. This kind of stress can be short-term, but it can be long-term if you keep on dragging it out.

KEEP CALM AND ...

The best way to boost your discipline and mental toughness is the ability to remain calm. This chapter will be dedicated to helping you keep a calm mind so you can achieve a new level of mindfulness that is essential. The calmer you are, the more disciplined you will be. Your levels of calm will also be a barometer for your mental toughness overall.

We'll show you ways to relax, how you can incorporate meditation, and how to become more mindfully aware of yourself at all times. This is a chapter you really should not skip (and for good reason). Without a calm mind, you'll be stressed all the time. And you'll allow yourself to apply more pressure than you already need to. Those who are undisciplined and not mentally tough will crack at a moment's notice.

By the end of this chapter, you'll have a few tricks up your sleeve on how to keep calm and carry on as they say. Doing so will help you achieve as many personal victories as you can. Let's dive right in and begin this chapter talking about relaxation.

RELAX

It's important to know how to relax. When you relax, your body won't feel as tense. Internal organs like your heart and lungs won't work too hard because you are not under amounts of stress. People tell us to relax like they know a thing or two. Maybe they do. But the reality is telling ourselves and others to relax is easy enough. It's the actual doing that can be difficult for many.

Relaxation techniques are much needed for a lot of us who face stressful situations on a regular basis. You'll learn a few of these in this section and find out why they are important. Some of these techniques will be your "go-to" options. If you keep doing them consistently, you'll be able to perform them like it's second nature. Here are some of our favorite relaxation techniques that we recommend:

Write it down: Keeping a journal is highly suggested. Especially when you want to develop discipline and mental toughness. In this instance, you want to write down what's bothering you. Take your thoughts and issues and put them to the paper (or in a Word doc if that's your thing). Take a few minutes out of the day to write out what comes to mind. What's bothering you? What can you do to solve the problem? Just you and your thoughts. No one but yourself will see it.

Just breathe: Later on in the chapter, we're going to go over a few breathing exercises. Having these on hand will really separate you from the pack. You can take a moment to find a quiet space so you can perform these breathing techniques. They can be in your workspace, in the bathroom, or someplace quiet where no one can bother you.

Make a gratitude list: Write down as many as five things that you are thankful for. This can be done in a daily journal entry or in a separate notebook. When writing down the things that you are grateful for, your mind is drawn back down to Earth. You'll come to the realization that you're thankful for what you got. Plus, it allows you to mentally focus on the positive as opposed to the negative.

Stretch it out: Stretches are one of the best ways to keep the muscles free of any tension. This can be basic stretches. Or you can take it a step further and do some yoga (which we will talk about later on in the chapter). Relaxation is mostly mental, but there are some physical aspects to it as well. Remember, stress can not only take a toll on you mentally but also physically.

Take it outside: It can be a nice sunny day outside and a bit warm as well. Sounds like the perfect day to go for a walk and get some fresh air. It's one of the perfect environments where you can relax and enjoy yourself. If you live in an area that is cold during the wintertime, you can take walks if you bundle up and can handle the chilly temperatures (but keep it short).

Relaxation gives you plenty of benefits. One major benefit that we're aiming for is the ability to think clearly and make better decisions without involving a high level of emotion. You can be able to solve problems with ease when you can think clear thoughts. You'll be able to get a 10,000-foot view of what decision will be the better of the two. If they are tough with some negative results at either end, you'll take the time to assess which option will yield the lesser amount of "pain".

As mentioned before, your physical health will benefit. When you're relaxed, you'll be able to enjoy health benefits such as keeping your blood pressure at lower levels. You'll also reduce your risk of heart attacks and autoimmune illnesses. Relaxation is good for the body and mind. There's no better way to say it.

CONCENTRATION

Knowing how to concentrate (even when it's "on demand") can be tricky. When you need to perform tasks that warrant your full undivided attention, concentration will be hard to come by. Lucky for you, we have some tricks up our sleeve that will help you acquire a new level of concentration that your friends and colleagues will envy you for.

When you have an improved level of concentration, you'll easily find yourself "in the zone" and get the tasks done. Wasting time will be the last thing you'll ever think of doing. In this section, we'll show you tips on how you can improve your concentration and focus. Along with that, we'll show you some of our favorite exercises that are guaranteed to help you concentrate even on the days when things can get very hectic.

Once you are able to concentrate and focus with the help of these exercises, you'll seem unstoppable. And you'll be able to keep the momentum going even on days when the daily task list is building up.

9 TIPS ON IMPROVING CONCENTRATION AND FOCUS

Without wasting any more time, let's take a look at the nine tips that you should take to heart when it comes to improving concentration and focus:

1. Get rid of distractions

As if this wasn't said enough times. Distractions kill concentration and focus in an instant. At this point, you should have a good idea on how to get rid of them. If you seem to experience a "slip of the mind" (don't worry, it happens), then go back to Chapter 3 where it talks about distractions and how to minimize them.

2. Focus on one thing at a time

Sure, people will brag about how they are the best multi-taskers in the world. We probably envy them. However, it's not smart to try to keep up with them. Sometimes, those who brag about being great multi-taskers can get into even bigger messes. But not you, though. You can focus on one thing at a time. When you focus on a single task, the quality and performance will be much better.

3. Take stock of your mental focus

Assessing your mental focus doesn't take a lot of time and effort. But you'll be able to know the difference between having it and lacking it. If you lose track of what you're doing or get easily distracted, it's clear that you'll need to work on it. If you manage to stay alert and take short breaks without dragging it out for too long, your mental focus should be right where it's at.

4. Be in the moment

When you're in the moment, you'll focus better. You don't focus on the past or the future. You are focusing on right now. In fact, consider the "past" and "future" things as glorified distractions. Don't worry about the "what ifs". Don't focus on past failures that will throw you off your game. When you tune your mind out of those things, you have no choice but to focus on what's right in front of you.

5. Take a short break

Sometimes, you deserve a break from what you're working on. You don't want to overwork yourself to the point where your focus and concentration evaporates. If you use a timer or use the Pomodoro technique, set a timer for how long you want to perform your task. After time runs out, take a short break ranging from 10 to 15 minutes. Once you allow yourself to re-group mentally, pick up where you left off. Also, resist the urge of getting too distracted on your breaks. A 15-minute break could stretch out to 30 minutes (which could get stretched to an hour).

6. Do light, physical activities

Tying into number five, you should use your break time as the perfect opportunity to do some light physical exercises. This can be a brisk walk around the block or finding a place to pound out some sit-ups and pushups. Or maybe there's a flight of stairs you can climb up and down to keep yourself in shape. You can keep your body and mind in good shape all at the same time. All it takes is 5 to 15 minutes.

7. Exercise your mind

Think that physical exercise is enough? Well, it wouldn't be fair to leave your brain out of the mix now, would it? Exercising your mind and keeping it strong will definitely help with concentration and focus. You can consider doing tried and true methods like crossword puzzles or similar games that you'll find in newspapers or booklets. Before you say anything, those brain games that you see online and on mobile apps may be fun to play. However, the jury is still out on whether or not they are beneficial to improving your focus. So, err on the side of brain exercises that don't require a lot of technology.

8. Don't TL; DR

You see that TL; DR all the time online. "Too long, didn't read" has become the norm for most people these days. So, most people would rather go for the executive summary of things rather than read it as a whole. But those who decide to read, and study lengthy pieces of writing will have more of an edge in terms of focus. Not to mention, it will help train your mind to absorb more information like a sponge.

9. Always keep practicing

Improving your focus and concentration is not some one-off thing. You do it over and over again. That's why it's always important to have a plan. Take regular breaks, reduce distractions, focus on one thing at a time no matter how long it takes. Practice does make perfect. And it will also help you become more in tune and focused compared to most people.

These nine tips will be helpful in making sure that your brain is on the right track when it comes to concentration and focus. Being able to deal with less distractions while focusing on just one single task are just two of the things you have to incorporate in your life if you want to make improvements. But that doesn't mean you have to ignore the other tips listed.

BE MINDFUL AND DEVELOP AWARENESS

Mindfulness is talked about a lot lately. However, a lot of people don't seem to get the message. Mindfulness is helpful whenever you want to develop a new level of self-awareness. Self-awareness is the ability where you know what you're doing. And it can be helpful in catching yourself when you're doing things that may be considered distractions.

We'll be taking a look at ways where you can develop mindfulness every single day. Not only will you be able to stop for a moment and gather your thoughts before continuing forward, you'll be able do this "on demand" whenever it seems hard to come by. Here are some things you'll want to do:

Practice mindfulness the moment you wake up: Being able to practice mindfulness the second you wake up is a must. It can be a quick five-minute meditation before you move on with the rest of the day. If for some reason you find yourself falling back asleep, you may want to consider drinking a cup of coffee or caffeinated tea before you do your mindfulness exercise.

Pay attention while doing routine things: As ridiculous as it sounds, paying attention to how you do routine things will help open up a part of your brain that is not often accessed because of our brain's "autopilot" feature. Focus on the sight, sound, taste, and feel of the activities that you normally do. Your autopilot feature will blunt these senses. But if you really focus on them, you'll probably uncover some interesting things about them.

Keep your mindfulness sessions short: Short mindfulness sessions will help keep your mind sharp and flexible. You can start out by doing a five-minute interval. Work your way up to 15 minutes max. Don't go any longer than it has to be. When you have short mindfulness sessions, it's a lot better than taking a week off just to relax.

Practice mindfulness in some stressful situations: When things get stressful, our brains get cranked into overdrive. While most will focus on taking out their frustrations on something or someone, you'll be a step above them. If you're waiting on the phone for a lengthy period (that on-hold music can be annoying), you can practice mindfulness exercises while you're waiting. The same if you are stuck in a traffic jam. Keep it short and sweet (as suggested in the previous tip) and stay in the moment. These stressful moments will pass whether you know it or not.

Meditation is your friend: Meditation is by far one of the best ways to achieve total mindfulness. Thankfully, we'll be talking more about it in the next section. Doing this on a daily basis will help you set the tone throughout the day. It can kill off any self-doubt and negative talk. Once you are present and able to keep a calm mind, you'll be saying things a lot differently. So instead of saying "this day is going to suck", you can say "this day will be stressful, but I have what it takes to handle it".

MEDITATE

Now, we get to the fun part. You cannot necessarily achieve complete and total mindfulness if you don't meditate. Before we go any further, meditation is not going to cause any kind of "depersonalization" or the like. But you'll feel like an entirely different person once you get the hang of it and experience some awesome short-term and long-term benefits.

We'll show you how to meditate the right way so you can do it for five minutes or even a half hour. Also, since meditation does require concentration, you'll want to pay close attention to these instructions. This way, you'll know exactly what to do without having to rely on written instructions. Alternatively, you can record the following steps below and put together a guided meditation.

Let's take a deep breath...and dive right in:

1. Get comfortable

First things first, you want to make sure that you are able to get comfortable. You'll also want to get it to a point where you can be able to sit still for a few minutes straight. At this point, the only thing you'll need to focus on is your breathing. In...and out.

2. Focus on the breath

At this point, you'll want to focus even more on your breathing. Where do you feel it the most? As you are breathing in and out (and continue to do so), see if you feel it most in your belly or through your nose.

3. Follow the breath

To do this, breathe in through the nose for as long as possible. As you do this, expand your belly. You can hold for a couple of seconds before exhaling slowly. Make sure the out breath is long and slow. Be sure to contract your belly while doing this. Start by doing this for at least two minutes and work your way up to longer periods whenever you feel comfortable.

And there you have it. You now know how to meditate in three easy steps. Pretty cool, huh? When you try this out, it will feel like an experience unlike any other. You might not get enough of it. However, you should consider doing this for a shorter period of time (even when done multiple times throughout the day).

BREATHE

Believe it or not, there is more than one way to breathe. In this section, you'll learn about some of the best tips about different breathing techniques and how you can do certain exercises whether you are sitting or laying down. Either way, this will help you get more in tune with your body so you can pay even closer attention to how you breathe.

Now, let's get you into becoming an "expert" on breathing. While most people will breathe on autopilot (because you have to), let's take a look at ways to control it so you are more in tune with your mind. Here we go:

The Navy SEAL breathing technique for maximum focus: If there is one more thing we can learn from the Navy SEALs, it's a breathing technique that will help them focus while they are on death defying missions. The first thing you do is breathe in slowly while expanding your belly. At the top of the breath, hold for four seconds. Exhale and contract your belly for four seconds. Then hold on the down breath for another four seconds and repeat the process.

Use your diaphragm to breathe: Remember when we said that you should breathe in and expand your belly? Well, keep doing that. Because you've just learned how to breathe from your diaphragm. Not only does this make breathing easier, but it also makes it less of a chore for your lungs to help you breathe. It will also strengthen your diaphragm in the process. Also, you may notice that your voice may become deeper or more powerful. That alone can make you more of someone who is viewed as authority. Just make sure you have the discipline and mental toughness to compliment it.

Do breathing exercises regularly: We'll be taking a look at two breathing exercises shortly. What you'll need to do is perform one of these for five to ten minutes per day. It's important to focus on your breathing and learn how to breathe from your diaphragm instead of breathing from your chest.

BREATHING EXERCISES TO TRY

We will be trying two different breathing exercises: one while you're sitting and the other while you're laying down. You can start out with either one of these. If you are a total beginner, try doing it for at least five minutes. You can work your way up to ten minutes if you feel more comfortable to make adjustments.

Let's start with the sitting down breathing exercise:

Breathing Exercise While Sitting

- Sit in a comfortable position. Make sure your knees are bent.
- Make sure you are completely relaxed. This includes your head, neck, and shoulders.
- Next, place one of your hands on top of your chest. The other hand will need to be placed below your rib cage. This will allow you to feel the movement of your diaphragm while you breathe.
- As you slowly inhale through the nose, make sure that your

stomach is pressed up against your hand. While doing this, make sure that your hand on your chest remains still.

- Exhale through your lips (while pursed). Make sure your hand on your chest remains still.
- Repeat the process for five to ten minutes.

Breathing Exercise While Laying Down

- Lie on your back with your knees bent. To ensure better support for your legs, place a pillow or two underneath your knees.
- Hand placement is the same. One on your chest and the other on you beneath your rib cage.
- Breathe in through the nose while your stomach presses against your hand. The hand on your chest must remain still.
- Breathe out the mouth (pursed) lips. Keep your hand on your chest still.
- Repeat the process for five to ten minutes.

When starting out, you'll try out both exercises to determine which of the two are the most comfortable. The laying down technique is slightly more difficult since you'll be on your back. Try each version once and decide which one will work best for you. As you probably notice, the technique is basically the same.

The main goal of these breathing exercises is to make sure you are breathing with your diaphragm as opposed to your chest. If the hand on your chest moves while you are breathing, you are not breathing through your diaphragm. It does take a bit of focus and practice to pull this off. And that's why we require you to practice this a few times a week.

Even after you are able to do this with little to no effort, it never hurts to keep doing it just to keep your breathing in check. Especially when you are meditating and keeping your mindfulness sharp.

THINK & DO ZEN

The focus of doing Zen is defined as centering your attention to the task at hand (which is basically what we're aiming to do). Believe it or not, Zen is a discipline. You don't have to be religious or commit yourself to Buddhism to know and use Zen to your advantage. Zen meditation is another opportunity to tune your mindfulness for the better.

But you can learn from the Zen discipline in order to achieve total mindfulness. You can meditate regularly. Focus on your breathing while clearing your mind. As mentioned before, Zen is all about discipline. It's about restraining yourself from what would possibly throw you off mentally and physically.

The Zen philosophy teaches you to be aware and in the moment. And when you are able to know that you're in the moment, the past and the future don't seem to matter. You'll be able to focus on the task at hand without caring about your past failures or worrying about future ones.

LEARN YOGA

Yoga is one of the best stress busters out there. Not only will it help improve your body physically, but it's also one of the best ways to keep your mind sharp so you are disciplined and mentally tough. While several schools of yoga exist, the concept is pretty much the same.

You can learn yoga by simply searching online for guides and videos on how to perform basic yoga poses. Also, if there's a yoga studio in your local area, be sure to see if there are some regular classes that are coming up. A basic yoga class might help in terms of helping you improve yourself in both body and mind.

BEGINNERS POSES YOU CAN TRY OUT

If you are a complete beginner at yoga, we'll show you a few poses that you can try at home. These are easy to do, and they won't cause you to twist and tie yourself up like a pretzel. You can do these anywhere as long as you have enough space and have a place where no one can bother you. Alternatively, you can get a few people to do some quick yoga with you so they too can beat the stress that gets thrown at them during the day.

Let's get right to the list:

1. Mountain pose

The mountain pose is the basic yoga pose. It's so simple that anyone can do it. What you need to do is stand up straight with your feet together. Your arms should be to your side. So, in other words, you're basically standing.

However, we're not done yet. Next, you want to squeeze your quads, so your kneecaps are lifted. You'll also want to draw in your abdominal muscles while lifting your chest and pressing down your shoulders. Also, try to put your shoulder blades as close together as possible. Make sure your palms are facing inward and lift your head up as if it's being pulled by a string. Hold this pose for five breaths (work your way up to eight breaths when you become more comfortable).

2. Plank

The plank is the perfect yoga pose whenever you want to work on your balance. While it's a simple pose, it's a bit physically challenging. In order to do this, get on all fours. Assume the "up" position as if you're about ready to do a push-up. Pull in the lower abdominals and pull the shoulders as far from your ears as possible. Pull in your ribs and hold the pose for five breaths.

3. Tree

This one requires a bit more balance. But unlike the Plank, you'll be in a standing position. However, here's the challenge: you'll need to stand on one foot. It doesn't matter which one. Lift one foot and cross it over the leg like you are making a "4". Stay standing in that position and hold for five breaths.

4. Child's Pose

For this last pose, this one will work to perfection whenever you need to get rid of tension and stress. What you'll need to do is get on your knees and lean forward so you are in a prone position. Tuck your knees into your chest and stomach. Then stretch your arms forward. You can allow your head to touch the floor or elevate it with a pillow. Hold the pose for as long as you like.

These are just a sample of the many poses that exist in yoga. But these four are the basic ones you can try right now if you like. Also, you should use a yoga mat whenever you want to try out these poses. That way, you won't have to rely on a floor that may be dirty or disgusting.

RECAP

Being able to keep calm and relaxed is all part of being disciplined and mentally tough. Especially when you want to achieve a high level of mindfulness. Mindfulness isn't just meditation alone. It can be focusing on routine things and going past your autopilot to really get a feel of the senses that go into things like brushing your teeth.

Meditation is important and you should do it for at least a few minutes a day. Not only will it allow you to clear out any stress and tension you may have, it will help you get through the day even when the going gets tough. Also, it wouldn't hurt to do some breathing exercises so you can be able to breathe through your diaphragm more and less with your chest.

It's important to instill some kind of discipline the same way those who practice Zen do. You can do this without being spiritual or converting to the Buddhist religion. The Zen philosophy has a ton of examples that will help you on the journey towards complete mindfulness.

Finally, take some time out of your day to do some regular yoga poses. They don't have to be complicated. The basics will do just fine even when you're starting out. It's possible to become more mindful than you are now. Having this power will separate you over many others around you. Mindfulness leads to a clear mind, better decision making, and handling almost any stressful situation.

BREAKING OLD ROUTINES AND CREATING EFFECTIVE HABITS

I f there is one tenant that is key to living a more disciplined life, it's all about adopting good effective habits. This chapter will be the ultimate roadmap towards breaking bad habits while instilling good ones in the process. It's true what they say: a bad habit is easy to form but very hard to break. With good habits, it's the other way around for most.

When the going gets tough and things get stressful, what bad habits are your go-to "comforts"? Do you smoke? Do you eat? What is your automatic response that stress can trigger? Or better yet, what is that trigger that will lead you to respond automatically to performing a bad routine you want to break.

You will learn how to form these good habits as if it were easy to do. Those who adopt good habits are usually more disciplined and mentally tough. Because their "can do" attitude will help them go from point A to point B no matter how long it takes. The debate about how long a habit can take to form is still debatable. But as long as you stay the course and form good habits (while watching your old routines disappear in the rear-view mirror, you'll be golden).

Now, let's finally say goodbye to those old habits that represent a lack of discipline and mental toughness:

THE STRUGGLE OF STICKING TO VALUABLE HABITS

Why is a good habit so hard to form? That's the million-dollar question. We may or may not finally have the answer to this question that has stumped many over the years. One of the main reasons why a good habit is so hard to form is because it's not as "attractive" as a bad habit. Attraction is not a word that ties into finding that significant other. Any habit that is considered "attractive" is something that will likely stick to a person for a longer period of time. Not to mention, the "reward" of exercising that habit will also further justify the decision to do it once (and then do it repeatedly when the need arises).

When there's a small region of attraction for a habit (like some good habits), then odds are the likelihood of that forming into something long-lived won't be good. In fact, it could have a 1 percent chance of surviving. However, there are ways to expand that region of attraction for good habits. That's performing the habit over and over again until it becomes a routine thing.

However, there's one thing to point out: someone who adopts a good habit expects to get it right on the first try. If they screw up, they throw their hands up and say "whatever, it was worth a shot". However, being consistent with a habit to a point where it becomes more attractive to do it because of the short-term and long-term rewards are what we're gunning for here.

For example, let's take a look at working out here. You know that the goal is losing weight. But you want to keep it as simple as possible. So, you purchase a kettlebell, learn a few workouts, and crank them out for about 20 minutes a day. You'll feel great, have more energy, and want to get it done the next time. No need to worry about "moving" parts or waiting for someone to leave the lifting station at the gym. If the conditions are right, you can form a good habit with little to no effort.

Why do you suppose we chose a kettlebell in this example instead of say regular weights? With a kettlebell, you just pick it up and start lifting. With regular weights, you have to walk to the plate rack, add the weights to the bar, lift, and so on. That may seem a bit complicated for someone, especially if they're actually crunched for time.

Also, one deviation from the initial conditions will also throw them off course. And that can throw a wrench into their plans of developing a good habit. When they see diminishing returns, they can either give up or level up. You can go from a 25-pound kettlebell to a 35-pound kettlebell or stop lifting altogether. What appears to be the best option for you in this situation?

Another key to forming a habit is repetition. You do the same thing over and over again. As tedious as it is, you keep doing it. The reward of being able to do the same thing without fail will help you form that good habit. Sure, there will be challenges and roadblocks. So, you must mentally expect them to happen. At the same time, it's important to stay focused and keep your eye on the prize.

DON'T RUSH! YOU CAN TAKE THE PATH OF SLOWLY BUT SURELY

Do you remember the legendary story of "The Tortoise and The Hare"? If you do, you know that "slow and steady" wins the race. Sure, the hare was fast and had an excellent speed advantage than the tortoise. However, the hare's complacency is one of the reasons why he lost. Meanwhile, the tortoise took his time and kept going.

The point is that when forming a new habit, it really doesn't matter how long it takes. But one thing is for sure, once you form a good habit you don't want to be complacent and forget about it. Also, you don't want to rush into forming a good habit either. Because the quality and longevity of the habit itself will be poor (and you'll fall back into old habits again).

Think about building a new habit like you're building a new skyscraper. It's a building that will change the city skyline for a long time. You are competing against a rival builder who wants to build a tower that is designed to be bigger and better. Your rival said that he can get it done faster than you (and you may not stand a chance to beat him). But you build yours anyways, brick by brick.

You are slowly but surely building the tower because the little things will add up over time. The building will get taller. And it will be more stable as it goes. You look over the little details and make some changes when necessary. When the building is finished, it stands strong and looks majestic. It may have taken a year to do it (which may not be the case for most habits), but the important thing was you took your time.

Meanwhile, your rival finished his tower in six months. He said he was going to get it done faster than you. Yes, it's bigger than yours. But it ain't better in terms of structural integrity. When a light wind began to blow, his tower began to crumble and collapse. Obviously, rushing into something will cause you to overlook some of the smallest possible details that are critical to forming a habit.

The moral of this story is that when performing the smaller tasks, it is less likely for you to resist the idea of doing it again and again. And that's the key to building a good habit. Where many fail to build a good habit simply boils down to getting the results fast and in a hurry. However, when they see that it's not like that, they call it pointless and give up. They need to accept the fact that it takes small steps or small blocks to build a good habit. And no matter how long it takes, they'll get there so long as they keep at it.

10 SIMPLE, YET INCREDIBLY EFFECTIVE, STRATEGIES FOR DEVELOPING POSITIVE HABITS IN ALL REALMS OF LIFE (IT'S MUCH EASIER THAN YOU THINK)

Below are ten of the simple and effective strategies to help you develop positive habits. These will be useful for all kinds of habits in every aspect of your life. Adopting these will make forming good habits a lot easier. People may envy you and some may even ask you "can you teach me how"? Either way, it's a good feeling knowing that you will be armed with a battle plan to form good habits.

Let's take a look at the first one:

1. Start out small

This can't be said better than this. Starting out small is a lot better than "going big or going home". It takes one small step to get started. It takes another small step to continue. Remember, small steps will likely get you to take another one. Don't feel like you have to make giant steps to go from one point to the next.

2. Set a small goal

Setting small goals will likely put you on the path towards forming a better habit. At the start, you should commit to 30 days to form a good habit. Some say it may be all you need to form a good habit to begin with. As we've mentioned before, the actual timing is a matter of dispute. A month may be easier to sustain for most. But if it's a bit of a challenge, you could get away with breaking it down to a smaller time frame like 7 to 14 days. After that time frame, reset the goal and do it again.

3. Remind yourself

Circling back to the last statement in number two, it's important to remind yourself to reset the timeframe that you set for forming a habit. So, if you commit to thirty days, set a reminder. When the reminder goes off, you'll know it's time to re-commit to another thirty and do it again. As tedious as it is, repetition is key in building a good habit.

4. Consistency is key

One of the true cornerstones of building a good habit is consistency. If you decide to work out for a span of 30 days, set an exact time on when to start doing it. 30 days of working out starting at 6AM will be the perfect recipe for building a habit. Because setting a specific time will be a "cue" to get you to act almost on autopilot. Speaking of which...let's talk more about "cues" or its original name in the next item on the list.

5. Form triggers

A trigger is defined as a ritual that you perform before you act on a certain habit. However, a trigger can be a set of conditions that will be perfect for a habit (good or bad). No matter how ridiculous it has to be (like snapping your fingers if you need a cigarette), a trigger will help you act on a good habit or break a bad one. As long as you follow through with it, you're golden.

6. Find a good replacement

If you are breaking a bad habit, then it's important to find something good to replace it. For example, if you are drinking soda but want to rely on caffeine to get you through the morning, consider replacing it with coffee instead. Remember to keep in mind the kind of values you want to retain (or risk losing) when breaking a bad habit and replacing it with a good one. If you place caffeine at a high value, don't deprive yourself of it when breaking that bad habit. There are more than enough ways to form a good habit while keeping your values intact.

7. Don't strive for perfection

As mentioned before, many people give up forming good habits because they expect to get it right and perfect the first time. Accept the fact that you will make mistakes and have a few stumbling blocks to cross over. What matters is that you keep going and correct any mistakes along the way.

8. Get an accountability buddy

Sometimes, relying on technology to remind you to keep going won't be enough. So, it's important to find someone you trust to help keep you accountable. It can be a parent, a sibling, or your best friend. Any one of these people who you highly value and trust are the people you want as an accountability buddy. It can be someone who wants to form the same good habits as you.

9. Eliminate the temptations

Are you losing weight but there is plenty of junk food in the cupboards? Throw them out. Are you spending money on something that isn't giving you a good return on investment? Cancel it. There are plenty of temptations that you can easily eliminate. Doing so will help you stay focused on that good habit without having to relapse bad into your old way.

10. Know the benefits

Knowing what the benefits are at all times will keep you going. It's also important to visualize what will happen if you stick with it (while doing the same in terms of what if you decide not to form a good habit). Where will you see yourself in six months to a year? Will you be feeling better knowing you have a few good habits? Or will it be the same old, same old?

FIND 'POSITIVE BEHAVIORS' AND HABITS THAT YOU CAN ACTUALLY ENJOY AND LOOK FORWARD TO

Looking for positive behaviors and habits that you are more than looking forward to are what disciplined, and mentally tough people always do. For them, it's as easy and effortless like ordering their favorite pizza. We'll be looking at some of the behaviors and habits that most people who are mentally tough and disciplined perform very well. You too when you decide to take them on yourself.

Here are just a few of those habits that you'll see from those types of people (and what you will likely do as well):

Know the distinction between letting go and giving up

Letting go is not the same as giving up. Here's an example of that. Let's say your ultimate goal is to have a prosperous and successful career. You decide that being a doctor is that best course of action. After you go through your undergraduate studies and apply to medical school, you figured that it may be time to go through the motions once more. Then one day, you decide that maybe being a doctor isn't what you really want to do.

However, you've had quite a deep interest in law for years. You love talking about it and you obsess over Supreme Court cases of historic proportions. So, you decide to drop out of med school in favor of law school. This is an example of letting go of something, not giving up. You've just created another way to get to your ultimate goal while letting go of the old way.

Giving up is basically just dropping the goal altogether. See the difference?

They are in total control

Simple enough, right? Those who are mentally tough are in control no matter how chaotic the situation is. They don't focus on the things that are beyond themselves. Focus on the things you can control and worry less about the things that you can't.

Eliminate the things that have no impact or value

Again, another simple thing to do. If it's a waste of time or it provides a negative return on value, get rid of it. This includes cutting out toxic people, canceling subscriptions that are a waste of money, and eliminating things you don't seem to have the time to focus on anymore.

Focus on impressing yourself

This may sound selfish or arrogant. But focusing on impressing yourself is a lot better than trying to impress others (and come off as some try hard). Besides, why should you vie for the approval of others when you can focus on something that you yourself will approve?

MORE AND MORE PEOPLE ARE USING THIS SELF-DISCIPLINE AND HABIT-FORMING SYSTEM

Lastly, we'll be taking a look at a simple to use habit forming system that will help you become more disciplined and be able to form a good habit no matter what it is. Without wasting time, let's get right to it:

Identify the routine

There are three things to a routine: the cue, the routine, and the reward. If it's a bad routine, you'll need to consider what's causing you to act on it. Also, you'll want to identify the reward when the routine itself is completed. Keep in mind that the long-term effects of the rewards may not be as good as you think.

Identify the cue

What is that cue or trigger that is getting you to perform that routine. If you have more than one cue, write them down on a piece of paper. Is it a certain mood that triggers it? Is it a specific environmental condition (i.e.-- you're home alone)? What time is it? What is your current mood? There are various conditions and the like that will make up the entire cue.

When it comes to good habits, create a cue that will help you execute on it. If it's a bad habit, know what the cue is and isolate it. You'll know exactly what the causes are for these bad habits by time, behavior, and the like.

Know the rewards

If you are trying to lose weight, then you know that the reward is living a healthy lifestyle. But it goes beyond that. People like to go a little deeper in their thought process. A healthier lifestyle means more time with their families, living a long healthy life, and a chance to do the things they want to do even in their golden years. The rewards go a lot deeper than you think.

RECAP

Breaking old habits and forming new ones can finally be a lot easier. There is no need for you to make giant leaps or expect the perfect results on the first try. The key here is to start small and start slow. Never mind about the timing. Never rush as it will increase the likelihood of giving up on a good habit too early.

It's important to follow the simple and effective strategies of building a habit. That way, when there's a good habit you want to adopt, you can be able to get it done with ease. Plus, you'll want to instill some habits that are used by mentally tough and disciplined individuals. Knowing that you're in control and being able to distinguish between letting go and giving up among other habits will put you well above the others around you.

Finally, you can put together a simple formula that will help you form a good habit (while eliminating a bad one) simply by identifying the routine and cues. Plus, knowing what the rewards are and looking deep beyond them will be a key factor in deciding whether the habit is good enough to form or bad enough to make changes.

OVERCOMING PROCRASTINATION AND MAKING FRIENDS WITH TIME

P rocrastination is one of the worst habits that anyone can have. It's easy for us to put things off until later on in favor of things we actually enjoy. However, in reality procrastination will add more pressure on you when timing is certainly not a factor. The more you have to get done when it's so close to the deadline, the greater the pressure. And that could be enough to get you to crack under pressure mentally.

This chapter will show you how to overcome procrastination and be able to enlist time as your greatest ally rather than your worst enemy. The truth is, time can really do you a favor if you manage it just right. You'll learn time management skills that you can adopt as early as today. When it comes to discipline, managing your time wisely is one of the must-have skills that you have to have. Especially when you don't want to waste it.

If you are one of the many people who procrastinate and actually want to conquer it, then this is the chapter you don't want to skip. Let's do it now:

IT'S POSSIBLE THAT IT'S THE DUNNING-KRUGER EFFECT OR PERHAPS YOU'RE JUST BEING LAZY

What exactly is the Dunning-Kruger effect? To simply put it into easy to understand terms, it's when people who are deemed incompetent cannot recognize just how incompetent they are. The explanation can go on for a long time, but let's just say that what it boils down to is that people tend to overestimate themselves when it comes to their abilities. You could absolutely suck at something but declare yourself the best in the world (though your actions prove otherwise).

One of the key things that could be the cause of this effect is ego. Are critical tasks that need to be done too good for you? Do you think that you can't be bothered for doing such things that have to be done? The Dunning-Kruger Effect could play a role in procrastinating.

When they say, "I'll do it tomorrow", it's a veiled way of saying "I've got better things to do than that". They are well aware that a certain task is important. But the problem is they refuse to acknowledge the importance at all. The Dunning-Kruger Effect and procrastination do go hand and hand to an extent. Procrastinating on purpose is a prime example.

Laziness and procrastination are not the same thing. But they are similar for one reason: all it takes is a lack of motivation. The major distinction between someone who is lazy and someone who procrastinates is the latter has aspirations (which eventually don't get fulfilled). Laziness is inaction where there are no aspirations to speak of.

PRACTICING DELAYED GRATIFICATION IS DIFFICULT, BUT IT'S DEFINITELY WORTH IT

Delayed gratification is the act of waiting to get what you want. For as long as you have lived, you have already experienced it to some degree. One example is Christmas. The presents sitting under the tree cannot be opened until Christmas morning. You're excited to know what you're getting, but you want to open up your gift now rather than wait later.

Practicing delayed gratification may be hard to do. And it may be a true test of willpower. But the reward at the end when you finally open that Christmas gift is all the more satisfying. Most things are usually worth the wait. Practicing delayed gratification will improve your self-control by leaps and bounds. At the same time, it will also help you achieve your long-term goals much easier and at a quicker rate of speed (without rushing into things, mind you).

Remember that Marshmallow Test we talked about earlier in our chapter about willpower? This is a prime example of delayed gratification at work. It's better to wait for the reward (no matter how sweet and satisfying it is). Though the good feeling of enjoying something may be tempting enough for you to act quickly, it all comes down to disciplining and restraining yourself.

Good things do indeed come to those who wait. But at the same time, those good things will also go to those with the self-control and patience to work hard and keep their eye on the prize. If you practice this, time won't be so much of the evil villain some people make it out to be.

THE POWER TO OVERCOME COMPULSIONS AND TURN AWAY WHEN FACED WITH TEMPTATIONS

Compulsion and temptation is a two-headed monster that many will encounter, but only few will slay. Are you one of the few to do that? First and foremost, let's define both compulsion and temptation. A compulsion is the irresistible urge to act a certain way while temptation is the desire to do something, even if it's not the smartest thing to do. When the two are put together, then that's when the real disaster begins.

Compulsive activities such as gambling, shopping online, or the like may be an unwise thing to do even if you do too much of it. If a compulsive gambler is not playing his or her favorite games online or at a casino, they will feel uncomfortable. But they won't undergo any severe physical withdrawals or anything. However, a compulsive gambler will find themselves in a monetary situation that will be hard to get out of.

Acting on your compulsions will certainly lead you on the road to poor health or financial stability. That's because you have no control over it whatsoever. When there's a cue, there's a signal for you to "go". With temptation, you are aware that the opportunity to gamble or eat when stressed is there. But you are also aware that there's a choice between doing it or not doing it. Those who are compulsive in their actions don't even take one nanosecond to think about it. That's the major difference.

Keep in mind that when you are apart from the things you do on a compulsive level; it's not going to make you sick. No one has even died from being deprived of the compulsive habits that they have done. But those same compulsive habits can lead to poor health problems where your lifespan could be cut short. We're not trying to scare you, but sometimes the truth about such bad habits and behaviors can be hard-hitting.

How exactly can you place a firm grasp on compulsions and temptations. We'll show you how to avoid them before things really get out of control. Here's what they are:

1. Recognize your compulsive behaviors

The first thing to do is recognize what your compulsive behavior is. It's also a good idea to know why you act on this without even thinking. This will challenge you to identify the cues and triggers. You will find out exactly why you act on your compulsions. For example, compulsive gambling could be stemmed by the idea of placing a large risky bet with the chance of winning big. The desire to "get rich quick" and make your existing financial issues go away can drive that compulsive behavior. Think of the feelings and the desires that trigger these behaviors.

2. Be aware of situational selection

Situational selection is something we face every day. Especially in situations where we are hungry or thirsty. Either way, you are faced with plenty of options. Do you go for Burger King or Subway? Coke or water? Get the idea. At this point, you are aware of what you can choose to satisfy your hunger or thirst. However, one option may not be as good as the other. Recognize which option is better for you in terms of the short-term and long-term benefits.

3. Practice situation isolation

Let's say you're in a situation where the temptations will be quite high. If you can't get out of the situation, the best thing you can do is isolate the "temptation". For example, if you are at a party where they serve alcohol and you drink regularly (but play the role of designated driver), stay as far away from the bar as possible. Opt for options that are farther away from your temptations. While it may be hard to do, acting on the opposite of the usual is a lot more rewarding.

4. Know the difference between fun and compulsion

It's one thing to gamble for the fun of it. It's another to do it compulsively. The main difference is self-control. Too much of what seems to be a good thing will always be bad. There is no other way to say it. It's important to distance the fun things from the stressful situations and the like. People use compulsive behaviors to escape from stressful situations or life in general.

5. Find a way to distract yourself from a temptation

We know that we've come down hard on distractions in this book. However, there are times when distracting yourself from something can be a good thing. In this instance, we're talking about pulling yourself away from a temptation. In other words, find something that will reroute your focus on that one thing instead of something you are tempted to do. The more you're into this new distraction, the farther you will distance yourself from the temptation.

6. Find like-minded people who have conquered compulsion and temptation

No one knows about conquering compulsion and temptations better than the people who have done it themselves. It's important for you to seek them out and ask for advice. They will be happy to help you find your way to beating compulsions and temptations. They've been there and done that. The last thing they could ever do is refuse helping those who are going through the same issues they have had in the past.

7. Don't fight, evade

Whoever said that the best way to win a fight is to never get into one obviously got it right. This is true in the case of compulsions and temptations. You'll want to avoid the fight and de-escalate it as much as possible. It doesn't hurt your ego in any way. Fighting your compulsion and temptations will be a waste of time. But you can find a way to isolate yourself from them as far away as possible.

BREAKING THE CYCLE BY TURNING THE NEGATIVE INTO A POSITIVE

Now, you're going to learn how to turn your negative thinking into positive thinking. We have reached the point where negative thinking is pretty much a pointless task to someone who is more disciplined and mentally tough. Having the ability to think positively will help you instill a new set of beliefs. If you repeatedly say good, positive things about yourself then chances are you will absorb those positive beliefs. And it will show.

With that said, let's take a look at some tips on how you can be more positive instead of being negative:

Never play the victim and assume responsibility: These days, it's easy for us to play the victim rather than claim responsibility for our own actions. It's up to you to create your own life. Don't wait for a specific circumstance. You have the option to take action or sit on the sidelines.

Say more positive than negative: It's true that if you say things that are negative or positive, you become that. Say it again and again and it will be embedded in your brain. If you have a can-do attitude and speak the same language, you will slowly adopt a can-do mindset.

Accept that no one is perfect (and neither are you): Anyone who says they are "perfect" in every way is a liar. No one is. And neither are you. When you expect to be perfect but fall short of your own expectations, that will discourage you from being positive. Doing the best, you can is a lot better than doing nothing at all.

Assess what you are thankful for: Take a moment and write down five things that you are thankful for. Focusing on this will help instill positive thoughts in your mind rather than the negative ones.

Be able to catch yourself: Some people think negatively and will let it flow through them. However, if you are making the switch between negative and positive, catch yourself thinking or saying those things. For example, instead of saying "I suck" you can say "I'm not that good, but I know I can improve". Sound simple enough, right?

YOUR TIME IS PRECIOUS, DON'T WASTE IT

Without question, time is a valuable asset in our lives. We can invest in it wisely or waste it. When you lose time, it's gone for good. You can never recover it. But when it's used to your advantage, the return on investment will be even greater. With that said, saying that "you don't have the time" is not a valid excuse. That's just a veiled way of saying "I don't have my priorities in order".

Keep in mind that there are 24 hours in a single day. Everyone is allocated the same amount of time in a day. It's how you spend it that matters most. Or better yet, it's a matter of how you prioritize your time. You should invest your time in things that you consider a high priority. The truth is, time can be taken away from anyone at any given time. The average person lives to be roughly 74 years old. People can live longer or shorter than that. That's why you should never underestimate time in the slightest.

That's why it is important to say "no" to the things that are a waste of time. It's better to invest time in getting the critical tasks done. When you do, you get a vast return on investment that can be spent on whatever you want (such as spending time doing the things you enjoy the most).

Unless someone invents a time machine or turns a DeLorean into one, we will never be able to turn back time. Spend it wisely or don't, the choice is yours.

TIME MANAGEMENT STRATEGIES THAT WILL CHANGE THE WAY YOU LIVE YOUR LIFE

Now, we'll be taking a look at some of the time management strategies that have long been tested and proven to work. Managing your time wisely will be key when it comes to instilling self-discipline in yourself. By the time you learn these strategies, some of these will stick out in more ways than one. You can even use one of these to help you invest more of your time in the important things rather than something that will give you a negative return.

Here are the time management strategies that you want to try out for yourself:

1. Plan and prioritize

As mentioned earlier, the excuse of "not having the time" is translated as "not having your priorities in order". You want to put the most critical tasks of your day up front every day before working on other tasks. That way, you invest in the true priorities that matter most. This can take some time. Especially when you are learning to recognize the real priorities from the ones that don't need a lot of focus at the moment.

2. Begin the day with a clear focus

When you get up in the morning, the last thing you want to wake up to is having your mind racing with seven billion different things. You want to wake up with a clear focus on what needs to be done today. You've already planned it the night before. Now, it's time to act on it. Focus on one thing and then switch to another when the task is done.

3. Eliminate procrastination

Obviously, procrastination is the enemy of time management. If you are going to say you're going to do something, you do it. Be someone whose words are like iron. Make it firm by doing what you say you are going to do. To say that you're going to do something, but never doing it will make you look bad. The sooner you get it done, the better.

4. Don't worry about multi-tasking

Multi-tasking can actually do more harm than good (contrary to what everyone else is saying). Simply put, focusing on one thing at a time and investing your time in that will definitely put you a head above shoulders over those who claim to be the world's greatest multi-tasker.

5. Recognize and minimize potential interruptions

If you are aware of some of the interruptions that may throw you off your game, identify them. Next, you want to distance yourself from them as much as possible. If checking your email or social media while in the middle of something is what you do, try to stop doing it and wait before you are finished with the task you're working on.

6. Split up larger projects

If you have a large project that can't get done in a day, it's better to break them up into small pieces. They can be split up into the tiniest of fractions. Day by day, hour by hour, and so on. The last thing you want to do is take on a gargantuan task and take as little breaks from it as possible.

7. Delegate any tasks that you can't work on

Is there something you can't focus on? Is there something that you can't do because you don't know how? The answer is simple: delegate. When you delegate tasks, it will alleviate any pressure you may have on yourself. Give the task to someone who is knowledgeable enough to get it done.

8. Rest and recharge

Resting up and recharging your batteries to do it all over again is essential. Without a good night's rest, you won't be able to focus on the tasks at hand the next day. Don't take all night and sacrifice sleep because something has to be done. Everyone has their limits...even you.

RECAP

Time management is easy to do now that you know how to get it done. Procrastination can exist in the form of the Dunning-Kruger effect or a lack of capitalizing on your aspirations. Procrastination should not be considered a form of laziness since those who are lazy lack aspirations. When reaching your goals or completing the tasks that will reward you, you'll feel a sense of satisfaction like no other. But when the timing is longer than usual, that can trigger delayed gratification. You know that the rewards are satisfying, but you will wait a long enough time to earn it. Delayed gratification is a true test of discipline and willpower that you can pass with flying colors (you've already done it as a kid just days before Christmas, mind you).

Overcoming compulsions and temptations will require you to isolate yourself from them as opposed to fighting them. Identify the reasons why your compulsive habits exist and find a way to lessen its power, so you are not so easily pulled in.

It's also important to switch your negative thinking into positive. When you think positive, it will show in your mindset, your body language, your words, and so on. And remember that time is a precious thing that you cannot lose. Once you waste a second, you never will get it back.

Lastly, managing your time will yield tremendous results when done right. When investing in your time wisely, your return will be far greater. And it can be spent on the things you enjoy most.

IT'S WITHIN YOUR GRASP, LITERALLY

Being able to have discipline and mental toughness within your reach is something you want to acquire. For most, it's farther away from them with every passing day. At this point, discipline and mental toughness are literally right in front of you. It's like an opportunity that is waiting to be taken by the right person. And people will tend to walk past it like they never notice it.

In this chapter, we're going to talk about the endowed progress effect. We'll explain what it is and how it pertains to discipline and mental toughness. When you are rewarded for your efforts and hard work, it's a good feeling knowing that you've started from point A and finished at point B. But what if you got something more than that? How would you feel if the reward was even greater than expected? Let's talk about that right now.

TRICK YOUR BRAIN USING THE ENDOWED PROGRESS EFFECT

The endowed progress effect is simply defined as receiving a bonus on top of your original reward for a job well done. For example, let's say you have a sales job and your goal is to sell at a rate of 20 percent. You successfully double the percentage and have a 40 percent sales rate. Not only are you rewarded for your normal payment, but you also receive a bonus for exceeding your goal.

Another example of endowed progress is a rewards program. Let's say your local coffee shop has a thing where you buy five coffees and get the sixth one free. Your loyalty to the business and buying the same item over and over again can give you a reward. It instills the reward that comes with the habit of coming into the coffee shop frequently.

When tricking your brain with the endowed progress effect, you are looking to work hard at achieving your goal and earning a much greater reward for completing it. That extra "reward" will motivate them to get the job done even though they actually won't earn something on top of the original reward in the end. Also, the endowed progress effects gets people to think that they have a head start towards completing the tasks at hand.

With that said, it's important to get a head start on achieving the goal. On top of that, using abstract measurements to track your progress will help you stay the course and complete the goal you are focusing on. Also, you want to focus on the time you already spent as opposed to the time you're about to invest in. That will give you the mentality of "I put this much time in it, I might as well continue". Also, focus on what's left to do as opposed to what's already done. Transparency is key when it comes to getting the job done.

PRACTICE DISCIPLINE AND PRODUCTIVITY USING BULLET JOURNALING

If there is one thing that you should consider doing while on the path of becoming more disciplined and productive it is using a bullet journal. What exactly is a bullet journal? A bullet journal is used to track everything in your life both in the personal and business side of it. You can write down something like a "to-do list" or a list of weekly plans that you can write out and execute. You can also use it to track things like income and expenses throughout the week. It's a to-do list, financial planner, and corkboard all rolled into one. And putting one to good use can help you become more disciplined and more productive in your tasks. So long as you consult and update it on a regular basis, it will definitely help you out in the long run.

You don't have to make it a very creative bullet journal. It can be organized and to the point. That way, you'll find your to-do list for the week or find an item on the list that you can get done in the next day rather than two days out. Bullet journals are fun to keep up on once you are able to get the hang of them.

BE SMART IN USING YOUR SMARTPHONE

Sure, we've been hard on the smartphone throughout a good part of this book. But we don't want you to give up on it entirely. There are ways to rely on it. Especially in a way that will help you keep track of your progress and remind you to perform certain tasks. A smartphone can be useful in terms of education. Most people will reach for their smartphones to access something educational versus their desktop computer.

Not only that, but you can also use a wide variety of apps designed for many things like task management, keeping track of your daily and weekly activities and so on.

The advantages and disadvantages of using a smartphone

What exactly are the advantages and disadvantages of using your smartphone? While there are some good things about using your smartphone, we cannot forget about the not so good things about them. Sometimes they are useful and sometimes they can be a distraction. Let's look closely at each advantage and disadvantage:

Advantages

- You can keep in touch with friends and family via text, phone call, and social media
- Play games, music, and movies anywhere you go
- Be able to set reminders to perform various tasks using specific apps that you can download on your phone
- You have it on you in the event of an emergency
- You can check your bank balance to see if you have any money on you at any given time thanks to apps provided by your bank.

Disadvantages

- Can be a distraction during times where focus on a priority task is needed
- Increased use has been linked to loneliness and other mental health issues
- Can cause sleep deprivation due to the blue light emitting from the screen
- May cause a lack of awareness around you (especially in a dangerous situation).

While using your smartphone can work to your advantage, there may be times where using it may not be necessary. You can use it to help you form good habits (if it's used properly). It's all about self-control and being able to know your boundaries. You can use it in your free time once you have completed the tasks and priorities you have planned for the day.

ATTAIN EFFICIENCY WITH MORE RELIABLE APPS AND TOOLS

Now, we'll be talking about some of the best apps and tools that we believe are essential in keeping track of your activities while building discipline and good habits. These are apps you can download and access on your smartphone. Some of them can also be accessed on your desktop or laptop computer. Either way, you'll be within reach of most of these apps.

You can use these apps on a regular basis so you can stay focused and keep track on what you've accomplished and what is left to do. We'll also explain why these apps may be beneficial to you as well. Let's start with the first app on the list:

1. Todoist

If you are looking for the best app to help keep a to-do list well organized, look no further than Todoist. Whether you sign up via email or by using your Facebook or Google account, you'll have to set up your to-do list that you can get done throughout the day or week. You can add new tasks or cross them off the list just by a couple touches of your finger or by using the sound of your voice. Either way, it makes to-do lists very efficient.

The best thing about this app is that it tracks your "Karma points". For every task that you get done on time, you earn more points. For every task that is overdue or finished beyond the due date, your "karma" will take a hit. It's the perfect rewards system to have in place for a to-do list app.

2. SimpleNote

Do you like taking notes? Do you have an idea so awesome that you have to write it down before you forget? Either way, SimpleNote will help you keep everything tidy in one handy little app. If you hate note taking apps that are loaded with so many features, this app will be something you might enjoy. After all, you don't want an app that will be hard to navigate and has plenty of clutter.

Best of all, it's free to use and is compatible with Android and iOS

3. Habitica

If you enjoy playing RPG-like games, then we've got some good news for you. Habitica is the best habit building app that will give you game-like features that will help you build more good habits with ease. Want to quit a bad habit and switch to a good one? Set it and level up with each small task you accomplish. Like Todoist, it has a reward system that will work to your advantage every time you accomplish something by the deadline. It can also "punish" you for tasks that are overdue or completed late.

Another great thing we like is the community feature. You can connect with like-minded people who are trying to form good habits and cheer them on as they are en route to building better habits. There is no better way to form better habits faster than having a solid support system.

4. Google Tasks

If you are a fan of Google's myriad of apps, thankfully there's a task app just for you. One of the cool things about this app is that it does the prioritizing for you. If you have critical tasks that you need to accomplish first thing, the app will help organize it to where tasks with the highest priority are on the top of the list.

This will also sync with your Gmail account and will also be accessible across other devices. If your Google account is linked to your devices, you'll have access to your task list. Your Google Calendar will be automatically filled with these tasks on your to-do list. That way, you are pretty much reminded to get it done everywhere you go.

5. Zoom

This app has gained a lot of fame in the past year. Especially when COVID-19 had most people scrambling to find alternative ways to meet up without the in-person contact. Zoom is perfect whenever you are running a business, conversing with family, or when you are taking a class.

With high-quality audio and video calls, keeping in contact with the people who matter most is easier than ever. Will we see the rise of Zoom meetings as opposed to in-person meetings going forward? That's a possibility. Especially when it will also reduce commute times for most people.

6. Asana

We've already looked at apps that focus on individual tasks. But what about for small groups and teams? Leave that all to Asana. This will allow you to set up tasks for your team members and help them keep track of their progress. You'll be able to set and assign tasks, prioritize them by setting deadlines, and set specific details so everyone on the team follows along and does what is assigned to them. If you are looking for the perfect app that is easily accessible and great for keeping track of everyone's progress, Asana is the go-to app.

7. Cold Turkey Blocker

If you are looking for something that will reduce distractions while working on your computer, Cold Turkey Blocker will come in handy. All you have to do is program it to where it will "block" websites that will serve as your distractions (i.e. -- Facebook, Twitter, etc.). When this is activated, try and access Facebook or any website you choose to block. You won't get through it. All you need to do is switch it on or schedule the app on when to block the websites in question and you'll be in business.

RECAP

Discipline and mental toughness may be within reach even when you are working on bettering yourself. At the same time, you can keep track of your progress while using your smartphone. Your smartphone is not your enemy when you are using it for all the right things. There are advantages to using them, but keep in mind that there are disadvantages that may hinder your level of discipline and mental toughness.

Be sure to check out the many apps that will help you manage your time, keep organized, and stay on task throughout the day. The seven listed above are just a sample of the dozens of apps that are available to download on both your smartphone and your computer.

V

APPLYING DISCIPLINE AND MENTAL TOUGHNESS IN YOUR LIFE

YOU MUST UNSTUCK YOURSELF

One of the things that people say is "I'm stuck". Especially when they are trying to make a move from one point to the next. This chapter will show you how to make yourself "unstuck". We have reached the point that getting "stuck" is just an excuse for saying you don't want to get something done. Or perhaps you are waiting for something or someone to motivate you.

The truth is that those who stay stuck will never get anything done. We have a section dedicated to that and we'll dive into it shortly. As mentioned earlier in the book, when you intend to find motivation, it's mostly elusive. It's like a cat or a dog. It will come to you if it feels comfortable enough to approach you. As weird as it sounds, what we're trying to say is the last thing you want to do is "chase" motivation.

When getting the job done, you will know that motivation has arrived. There will be no stopping you when you start. If you are looking for a new way to obtain the motivation without even thinking about it, keep reading. This chapter will hand you the new way to get motivated (even if you've failed to find it in the past). Let's get going:

YOU DON'T FEEL LIKE DOING IT? THEN YOU'LL NEVER END UP DOING IT

Earlier on, we have said that the more you keep saying negative things, the more you will become it. This is such a case when you say, "I don't feel like doing this or that". For this reason, when you repeat this process, you develop this habit of not wanting to get anything done. So, you end up not doing it. This is one of the symptoms of procrastination or laziness (depending on whether or not you have the aspirations to do something).

People are looking for those "perfect moments" to get started on some task. Otherwise, what's the point in getting it done? Here's the thing: if you are looking for a "perfect moment", we can finally unveil it right here to the world. We're so excited we can't wait any longer. The perfect time to get started on something is...drum roll please...right now! Yes, there is no "perfect moment" better than right now to get something done.

Waiting for the perfect moment is a complete waste of time. And remember, the time you waste is the time you never get back. It's as simple as that. You can accept this fact and get started or you can be a prime example of the Dunning-Kruger Effect and be aware of that while choosing not to take action. Either way, the choice is yours.

Remember this age-old quote: "The best time to grow a tree was 20 years ago. The second-best time is now".

JUST GET THE BALL ROLLING

At risk of turning this into a physics textbook, we quote the following from Newton's First Law of Physics: "Objects at rest tend to stay at rest. Objects in motion tend to stay in motion". Obviously, the point is you need to get moving in order to get something done. There are some things that will obviously help you get the ball rolling. Clearly, motivation itself is not one of them. You need to find a starting point to ensure that you build up as much momentum as possible so you can move on from one task to the next with little to no issue.

Getting started on something can be as simple as visualizing the action itself and the outcome that follows. Think of the reward that you'll earn for a job well done. Also, think about what could happen if you don't get the job done? Visualizing it and incorporating the emotion within it may be enough to get the ball rolling.

Another thing is to program your mind into being in the moment. You can do that by focusing on the breathing techniques that we've discussed in the chapter on mindfulness. To have a clear mind that is laser focused on the now will help you achieve a focus like nothing else. When you are focused, that's when the ball moves. And when it moves, it keeps moving until the task is complete. But if it's a task that requires a lot of time, do part of the work, take a break, and keep going.

There are small tasks that you must complete before getting started. Get one out of the way, on to the next one. And so on. Remember, the small tasks will help you stay focused. And it's one step closer to getting whatever you need to finish said and done with. We guarantee you that you won't be overwhelmed in the slightest.

One thing to remember about motivation. It's not motivation that starts moving the ball. It's what keeps the ball moving. In other words, **motivation is momentum**. As long as you start with the vision of succeeding at your goals in your mind, motivation will find you when you keep going.

MAKE INFURIATING TASKS BEARABLE

In every task we perform or every job we work at, there is always one thing that we absolutely hate to do. For example, if you work at a convenience store, some of your tasks may include changing the inside and outside trash cans. Another task is cleaning the bathrooms. They are dirty jobs, but someone has to do them in order to keep the place clean. You'll notice that a lot of people hate doing the dirty jobs, so they shift the responsibility to someone else. Naturally, it may anger you.

However, it shouldn't anger you. It should give you the opportunity to prove yourself to others that unlike themselves, a task that is unbearable doesn't bother you in the slightest. Your boss may notice that and may praise you for it. The point is that not every person on Earth has the mental strength nor the positive frame of thinking to do the "dirty jobs".

But not every unbearable task has to be dirty. They do however require you to make decisions that could change the entire trajectory of someone's life or career. It could even change the path of an entire business. Sometimes, you will be faced with two decisions that will have negative results at the other end. And it will impact someone or something in a way you don't want to see. So, making a decision where the impact is not as severe is what you're gunning for. It's a decision that you don't want to make, but deep down it's the best course of action going forward.

Unbearable tasks can also be "boring" as well. One way to make them as less boring as possible is to find something interesting about the task. It doesn't matter how ridiculous it sounds. Plus, you don't have to share that observation with other people. Just find something that makes the task less boring to do. You can also use the opportunity of performing a boring task to sharpen your mindfulness. Feel the task, hear the sound of it, and make the smallest observations that no one seems to notice. It's a lot better than doing it on autopilot while grumbling about it, right?

IMAGINE THE FUTURE AHEAD OF YOU

Visualizing the future and what you can accomplish can help you drive yourself to start achieving the tasks at hand. Imagining a future where you are able to accomplish anything with little to no delay may just be enough for you to get the ball rolling. A fulfilling, positive future is what we aim for. We don't want to be stuck with the same old, same old six months or even a year down the road. While the future may be bright for us, you still need to focus on the now in order to see it in full view.

One of the visualization techniques that will work to your advantage when thinking about the future is known as the 10-10-10 rule. The way it works is this: Imagine a decision that you are about to make. It's something that will have some degree of impact over the course of time. What you want to do is visualize the decision as if you made it already. How will it impact you 10 minutes after the fact? How about 10 months? Now try 10 years?

It sounds like there is some kind of ripple effect that occurs with just one decision you've made. It can also have some kind of impact on the rest of the decisions and life events that will occur in the future. Especially the ones that will happen ten minutes from now. This is why visualization is so important. You can think about making the decision and think about how you feel about it.

In 10 months or 10 years' time, you'll feel like you could have done something different. Or you can feel good knowing that it was the right decision and you don't regret making it. Either way, it will have an effect on you long after you've made the decision yourself. Before making a vital decision, use the 10-10-10 rule to your advantage when visualizing what will likely happen once it's made.

The lesson here is that every decision will have short-term and long-term effects. Whether they will be negative or positive will depend on what you've decided on. If anything, this will give you a chance to ponder your decisions and choose the right one without hesitation.

PUSHING THROUGH, EVEN ON THE WORST DAYS

In life, there will be good days and bad days. And there will be the worst days of your life. Even on those days, it's better to get through them the best that you can. One of the caveats of pushing through on your worst days is that you still need to keep your limits in the front of your mind. You don't want to push yourself too far or it will have adverse effects on your health (both mentally and physically).

Working through your worst days will be one of the ultimate tests of your discipline and mental toughness. You will have negative emotions running through your mind. It's okay to be sad or angry about things. And remember, being mentally tough does not mean becoming an emotionless robot. However, you don't want your emotions to overcome you to the point where the decisions you make will be solely based on your emotions without a hint of logic. It will likely throw things off course.

Even on your worst days, the key here is to find the good among the bad. For example, what would happen if you just took a deep breath, took it slow, and gave yourself enough time to gather your thoughts and make an important decision that could affect your future? Things may turn out for the better because you gave it some thought rather than let your emotion cloud your judgement.

It's okay to make mistakes. It's okay to keep going when the day isn't going your way. All that matters is that the emotions of it all should not get to you. One thing that will make you feel better through all the bad stuff happening in one day is the positive feelings you'll get whenever you complete the tasks that need to be finished. You will feel a lot better in ten minutes after finishing it. Not to mention, you will feel good about it 10 months and 10 years afterwards. You will think back on that day and remember some of the positives that happened instead of the bad.

DOPAMINE CAN BE YOUR BEST FRIEND OR WORST ENEMY

Dopamine is the chemical in your brain that makes you feel good about things. It can be your best friend or your worst enemy depending on the situation (or the decisions you make). Either way, you need to frame your mind as to how dopamine can serve you best. When you are eating something unhealthy, dopamine is released to make you feel good about eating something tasty. But the reality is, dopamine in this situation is like that friend who will say things about loyalty and respect but turn around and stab you in the back years later. In this context, when eating junk food, you will suffer the long-term consequences such as weight gain and the potential health effects that go along with it.

You can also get a dopamine rush by doing something that will have a positive effect on you in the long run (especially for your health). It's about training your mind to release that dopamine whenever you do the right things. So how do you go about doing this? You could do what is known as a "dopamine fast". This could mean avoiding the usual activities that you do in order to make you feel good about it. This might mean eliminating smartphone use for a short period of time. Or it could mean not talking to people for a set time period (which may be risky for those who tend to be more social). It's about finding that one task that releases a good amount of dopamine and cutting that out of your life temporarily to reset your brain.

The jury is still out on whether or not it works. But you could try it for a short period like a week. After that period, you can decide to do it for another week. Do it until you feel that there is a shift in your brain where you can get the dopamine rush you need from the things you can get done as opposed to the things that make you lazy or inactive.

Even if you finish a task where you had a hard time getting started, the feeling of getting it done anyway will guarantee that dopamine rush. And it will be the first of many if you keep doing it.

RECAP

If you are stuck, the best way to get unstuck is to get moving anyways. There is no point in waiting for the right moment or searching for that motivation. You visualize the future of performing the task and what happens after that. Remember, every decision you make will have an impact on you ten minutes, ten months, and ten years from now. In those future time frames, will you feel good about it? Or will you wish that you took the action when the opportunity presented itself?

You will also be faced with tasks that no one will like to do. It's up to you to set the example that even though the task is not something you enjoy; someone has to do it anyway.

Visualizing the future will be key in accomplishing something. Especially if you are having the worst day of your life. There will be worse days. And it will be up to you to put your discipline and mental toughness to the test in order to get through them. You will feel good and have that moment of positivity once you get something done.

That rush of dopamine will certainly make you feel like the tasks you're supposed to do are effortless. However, the dopamine release can seduce you into making bad decisions only if you allow them to happen.

KEEPING YOURSELF FIT AND HEALTHY

While discipline and mental toughness will spread out through all aspects of your life, you should also remember to utilize it when you want to live a healthy and fit lifestyle. Sure, the road to living a life where you are healthier and in better shape will be a bumpy one. Yet, at this point you should have the awareness and knowledge that you will need to incorporate discipline and mental toughness to start the journey, continue on it, and get to the destination.

Every person has unique goals when it comes to living a healthy life. Some may want to lose 20 pounds while some will want to lose just 10 pounds. Either way, there is a goal out there that you can set and achieve. Plus, it will be a lot easier to get there as long as you are aware of any potential setbacks that may pop up out of nowhere.

We'll talk about discipline and how it should be as routine as brushing your teeth. We'll also discuss which exercise routine will work to your advantage. We'll also talk about other habits that will tie into being healthy and fit such as your diet and getting a good night's rest. While we are not fitness experts in the slightest, this chapter will save you a lot of time and will help give you a better understanding of how living a fit and healthy life ties in with discipline and mental toughness.

Keep reading if you are looking to make amends on your life when it comes to your overall fitness:

DISCIPLINE WILL MAKE MASTERING THE FUNDAMENTALS OF HEALTH AND HAPPINESS AS ROUTINE AS BRUSHING YOUR TEETH

The truth is, discipline will be one of the key building blocks in making sure that you stay on top of your health and fitness. It is important to instill self-discipline since it will help you make decisions with a better understanding of the consequences or results (depending on the magnitude of them). By this we mean the following: if you were hungry and had to choose between McDonalds and Subway, which one would you go with? On paper, the choice is obvious. Subway has much healthier options compared to McDonalds (despite the fact that the latter serves up salads as their only healthy option).

If you eat junk (albeit on a consistent basis), that will negatively affect your overall health and fitness. However, if you choose to restrain yourself from eating it and opt for something healthier instead, that's a good sign. Self-discipline is the ability to restrain yourself and give into the temptation of something that may taste good, but can really hurt you in the long run.

With discipline, you can easily say "no" to the junk food and yes to the foods that will help you build muscle, perform better in the gym, and ward off any ailments that can get serious in a moment's notice. Also, self-discipline will keep you on the right path in terms of how you use alcohol. Instead of binge drinking or getting drunk, you can use moderation. Self-discipline can also help you stay away from drugs, which some people will use to "escape" life in general.

With consistent self-discipline, you are less likely to make impulsive decisions. You will be able to think clearly and use your head when making a decision. Of course, impulsive decisions don't require you to think about your choices and actions. The deeper you embed discipline into your mind, the more routine it will become.

Discipline will help you set forth a routine that will ensure that you stay in shape for as long as possible. Imagine getting up in the morning and ready to do a quick one-mile jog before the day begins. Or getting out of bed, doing a couple sets of kettlebell swings and call it done in 10 minutes. With routine discipline, it will be like second nature.

YOUR DAILY EXERCISE ROUTINE

First off, your daily exercise routine can be done at a time of the day where there is a good amount of time to yourself. Usually it's in the early morning hours. For some, it can be later than that. However, the first thing you need to do before setting up an exercise routine is choosing the time block that works best for you. We have 24 hours in a day. There is at least a block of one hour that will be considered "free".

Remember, if you "don't have the time", you want to straighten out your priorities. So, what exactly is your daily exercise routine? Does it have to be at the gym? The good news there is you don't have to go to the gym in order to incorporate a daily exercise routine. It can be as simple as doing it at home using a yoga mat, a kettlebell, or both. You want your exercise routine to be as simple as possible (even if you do have a little bit of time on your hands).

The key here is that you want it not only to be simple, but it also requires small steps. Obviously, with fitness there will be times when you'll be doing the same thing over and over again. Three sets of 12 repetitions of one exercise (and the same for the other exercises you have planned out for the day). The more you keep doing it, the stronger and fitter you become.

SIMPLE EXERCISES TO TRY OUT

If you have never had a fitness routine before and want to start, we'll show you how to put one together with the help of these simple exercises we'll list below. Not only will you be able to choose a couple to start, but you can put one together where you can do a combination of a few exercises per day that focus on specific areas of the body.

Here are some simple exercises that you should consider trying out for yourself (even if you don't have a clue how to set up a fitness routine):

1. Lunges

If you are looking for an exercise that will help with balance and leg strength, lunges are one of the most reliable exercises around. To perform lunges, here's what you'll need to do:

- Stand with your feet at shoulder width and your arms down at the side
- Using your right leg, step forward and bend your knee. Stop when your thigh is parallel to the floor. Also, make sure your foot does not extend past your knee
- With your right foot, push off and return to the standing position. That's one lunge. Now, do the same thing but this time with your left leg.

2. Push ups

One of the most popular forms of calisthenics widely practiced today is push-ups. This will help with building upper body strength. Plus, there are some variations that you can try once you get the hang of them. But for now, let's stick to the basics. To perform push-ups, this is how you do them:

- Start in the plank position. Your body should be upwards with your arms in a straightened position
- Bend your elbows and lower your body down to the floor. Make sure that your chest barely touches the floor or at least an inch off of it. Make sure your elbows are close to your body when doing this

- Return to the plank position. That's one push up. Repeat with as many as necessary. You can start with five, ten, or fifteen. As you get the hang of it, you can try and perform as many until failure.

3. Squats

The good thing about squats is that you can do them with weights or just by using your own bodyweight. For the sake of keeping it basic, this and other exercises will require no weights. With that in mind, let's learn how to squat:

- In a standing position, make sure that your feet are a shoulder's width apart
- Take your arms and raise them behind your head. You can clasp your hands behind your head or raise your arms straight ahead at chest level
- Brace your core and keep your head and chest straight. Then lower your hips and bend your knees. The motion will be as if you are sitting down. Hold the down position for one second and return to the standing position. That's one squat
- Do as many squats as necessary or have a set number in place.

4. Burpees

Now, this is where things will get really challenging. And if you love challenges (you probably do at this point), you might want to give burpees a try. These may be the closest you can get to a full body workout (with a little bit of cardio involved). How do you pull off a burpee? Let's show you how:

- Start in the standing position with your feet at shoulder width
- Bend your knees as if you are doing a squat. Once you reach the low point, transition into the plank position and do a push up
- After performing the push up, return to the up position and jump up in the air. That is one rep
- If you are a complete newbie, perform three sets of 10 burpees. Make adjustments once you get the hang of it and want more of a challenge.

5. Planks

This may be one of the most challenging ab exercises there is, despite looking so simple to do. To pull off a plank, here's what you need to do:

- Get in position as if you are doing a push up. Or you can rest your arms on the floor while they are in a 90-degree position
- Hold the position and tighten your abdominal muscles. Hold for 30 to 60 seconds.

These five exercises are just a sample of some of the most basic exercises that you can do on a daily basis. You don't have to lift heavy weights to start off with building a reliable fitness routine that can be done almost every day. Also, it would be wise for you to choose a day to rest so your muscles can recover and recuperate.

YOU ARE WHAT YOU EAT

It's true what they say, you are what you eat. In this context, either you are healthy or unhealthy. So, what can you do to assume a healthy identity? Aside from regular exercise, having a healthy diet will be key to living a healthier and fit life. It's even more important to know some of the awesome benefits that eating healthy can provide.

All the essential vitamins and minerals, out there are linked to various health benefits such as strong bones, boosted testosterone levels, clearer skin, and many others. So, it's important to know what you're eating if you are shooting for specific benefits like reducing your risk of heart disease or cancers (especially if it runs in your family).

With the right amount of whole grains, fruits, and vegetables (among others) as part of your diet, you'll be eating a lot healthier than most people. If you are planning on eating healthy, consider adding some fresh fruits and vegetables from the produce section to your shopping list next time. Also, opt for whole grain bread instead of white. Also, you should consider choosing fat-free or reduced fat options for most foods.

IMPROVING YOUR OVERALL HEALTH

Believe it or not, self-discipline is a lifesaver. It will improve your overall health in both the physical and mental sense. If you are not at a level that you are satisfied with, it's important to consider making improvements now rather than later. The first thing you should always do is consult with a doctor. You can start by scheduling a checkup (which should be done every year). Your doctor will be able to assess your health and help you get on the path to a healthy lifestyle. If there are some health issues that are discovered, your doctor may recommend medications or other alternatives to treat it.

If you are dealing with health issues that are mental, there is no shame in seeking help from a professional in the mental health field. It can be a therapist or a psychiatrist. This way, you can talk to someone about your problems. Do not worry, everything is kept with strict confidentiality. But keep in mind that it is okay to talk to someone who you trust whenever you are dealing with mental health issues. Also, keep in mind that you can still acquire mental toughness and discipline even if things aren't going right mentally to begin with.

HOW MUCH SLEEP WILL AFFECT YOUR WHOLE DAY?

They say that you need 7 to 9 hours of sleep per night in order to fully function. The truth is a good night's rest will be beneficial in the way you focus. Not to mention, it's healthy for you to get a good night's rest. When you get the proper amount of sleep, you will wake up refreshed and with an easier ability to focus and use that energy to get the day's work done.

But getting a good night's sleep isn't just for focus. It will also help when you want to improve your physical fitness altogether. When sleeping, your muscles will repair faster and will aid in strengthening them. Plus, those who get a consistent amount of sleep on a nightly basis will be less likely to consume more calories throughout the day. So, it will make weight loss a lot easier for most. Those who sleep poorly will tend to eat more throughout the day.

RECAP

Discipline is one of the cornerstones towards living a healthy and fit lifestyle (both mentally and physically). Not only should you keep yourself in good physical conditions, you should also adopt a diet that will help complement that healthy lifestyle. Even if you have never done any exercises, you can try out some of the basics listed in the chapter.

You are what you eat in terms of your overall health. So do your best to change that if you are eating foods that are not good for you. It's fine to treat yourself so long as it's in moderation. But eating a healthy diet where you get plenty of vitamins and minerals will yield its rewards for the long-term.

Improving your overall health can start by visiting a doctor and maybe a mental health professional (if you are dealing with mental health issues). These are people who live to help get people on the right course so they can live healthy and more fulfilling lives.

CONCLUSION – THINGS THAT YOU SHOULDN'T FORGET

Before we wrap things up, we're going to go over a few things that you shouldn't forget. First off, let us remind you that this book is not one of those "one and done" books. We encourage you to keep this book on hand so you can use it as a reference guide. Building discipline and mental toughness will take time. And you will need something to fall back on in case you are stuck with something. This book will always have the handy instructions that will get you unstuck.

Your journey towards discipline and mental toughness will be one of the most interesting and challenging things you've done in your lifetime. But rest assured, the rewards at the other end will be even sweeter. You will live a fulfilling life where you can get the tasks done at a moment's notice and say "no" to the things that will distract you.

Now, let's take a look at the four major things you should not forget to do:

ALWAYS DO MAINTENANCE

Maintaining your discipline and mental toughness will always need to be done. Just like building your muscles, you want to maintain them regularly by eating a protein-rich diet and working out regularly. What are some of the best ways to do maintenance? First, you should keep track of everything and look over the data again and again. How often are you meeting your goals? How long is it taking you? Is there any data that will point to you making changes and improvements?

Also, you shouldn't take your support network for granted. You should do your best to keep in touch with them and lean on them in times where you feel unsure or stuck on things. They will give you advice, encouragement, and remind you that no matter what, you have what it takes to get the task done. If there are those in your network that tend to be more negative than positive, then it is your responsibility to find a suitable replacement while eliminating the toxic attitudes within your support group.

Your support network doesn't always have to be your most trusted friends and family. It can be like minded individuals online who share the same goals and aspirations as you do. Either way, you'll always have people to turn to when the going gets tough.

One of the last building blocks to maintaining discipline and mental toughness is being persistent. In other words, you keep going. You keep the momentum going no matter what stands in your way. Imagine being a speeding train with no brakes. There are brick walls in the way. And you are going at such a fast rate of speed that those walls don't stand a chance. You bust through them and keep speeding onward.

YOU'RE NEVER ALONE

Of course, you're not the only one that is traveling on the journey. Without them, you won't have a support network of like-minded individuals to turn to. There are more people than you realize that want to instill self-discipline and mental toughness. The good news is, there will be a handful of people who will achieve success. The not so good news is some of them will do a few more attempts before finally being able to get it done. It doesn't matter how long it takes for someone to develop discipline and mental toughness. As long as you're doing it, you'll be just fine.

However, the thing to know is that it can get lonely up at the top. That's because there are many people who will start trying to attempt an ultimate goal. But few will actually make it. Even though the top has a few people, you'll feel alone and feel like you're the only one who has made it. But don't let that thought incorporate any negative feelings. You can still be able to connect with the like-minded people who made it alongside you.

As mentioned before, your support system will also help you become more disciplined and mentally tough. You will always have people to turn to when you have questions to ask or if you are struggling with something. Remember, there is no shame in asking for help. And you should never be too proud to reach out for help. Just know that your support system will always be there whether you are starting from zero or have already become more disciplined and mentally tough.

REMAIN HUMBLE AND COMPASSIONATE

When people finally achieve some kind of success, it's common to see them change in terms of their behavior. When someone wins the lottery (for example), they could let money easily change them and therefore behave in a way where it could affect personal relationships. In short, people who find success will often let it go to their head. They may start acting superior and think they are better than everyone else. The truth is, they are lacking in discipline and humility. Sure, they may have mental toughness. But that's only a facade that can come crumbling down.

When you reach new heights and success in your life, it's important to remain humble and compassionate. Even if you are disciplined and mentally tough, it's always a good idea to remember those who have helped build you up. You will need to give credit to those who have been able to stick with you from day one and beyond. When you are mentally tough and disciplined, you will still need to show compassion for those who may be struggling to achieve their goals (or with life in general). You don't have to help everyone in distress. But you could do your best to point them in the right direction if asked.

Humility will allow you to never lose sight of what you are thankful for. With discipline and mental toughness, you will likely be more compassionate because you have dealt with your own struggles in the past. And you may be the person that helps that person out. Whether the other person accepts that help from you or not is entirely up to them, so don't force it.

There's a good chance that you come from humble beginnings. And you have a better understanding of what it's like to have nothing. Do your part to listen to those who are struggling and help them solve the problem. You may not need to solve it yourself. But you may know someone who will. Also, it won't kill you to be a part of someone's support network as well.

REWARD YOURSELF

Of course, you deserve to reward yourself for all the hard work you have accomplished. When it comes to building up discipline and mental toughness, it's a good idea to reward yourself after you've reached an important milestone. Even the smallest of steps made deserve a bit of reward. If you want to move onto the next task with little to no effort, it's better to reward yourself so you can continue on.

The bigger the tasks, the sweeter the reward. It's kind of like the old "carrot on a stick" trick. With the carrot dangling in front of you, you can be the rabbit that chases after it. Only after a certain period of time where you have accomplished the tasks that will inch you closer to the goal, will you enjoy that carrot for yourself.

Also, you'll want to remember that there will be times when you miss doing a task by accident. It may happen due to forgetfulness. The important thing to do is not be hard on yourself. It's easy to do that when you make a mistake that's trivial and not so much a big deal. So, if you goof up, just accept it and move along. Just remind yourself that it's okay to make mistakes. True discipline is restraining yourself from being negative both in your thoughts and in what you say to yourself.

RECAP

When it comes to discipline and mental toughness, it is better to build it up and maintain it throughout your entire life. The old "set it and forget it" philosophy won't work as it will develop complacency and wipe out all the progress that you have worked on. It's hard work, but it will be a lot easier to maintain it throughout every day of your life.

Another thing to keep in mind is that you will never be alone on your journey. There will be like-minded individuals who will share the same goals and aspirations as you do. They will face similar challenges. And they will see to it that they will fulfill those goals come hell or high water. These people can also become a support network separate from the one that consists of your close friends and family. You won't feel alone on your journey, even though there may be less people at the top of the mountain.

When you finally achieve this success, the last thing you want to do is let the success go to your head. Considering that you have started from zero and understand the struggles of having a lack of discipline and mental toughness, retain that humility and compassion so you can use it as a way to position yourself as the person who has been there before. Especially when you are helping someone out.

Finally, rewarding yourself is key when you want to keep going with achieving the goals you have set. Reward yourself whether it's the little things or when you've reached an important milestone. It is the rewards that will keep you moving forward. And before you know it, it's mission accomplished.

OVERCOME PROCRASTINATION & OVERTHINKING (2 IN 1)

DEVELOP YOUR SELF-DISCIPLINE, MENTAL TOUGHNESS, & HEALTHY LIFELONG MINDFULNESS HABITS TO FULFIL YOUR POTENTIAL & SMASH YOUR GOALS

INTRODUCTION

It's something most of us do every day and throughout the day, often without even knowing it. It has roots which reach out across our lives, from the deepest core of our minds and bodies through to the people around us and then even further, to the ends of the Earth and even beyond.

Procrastination and overthinking may not seem like a global pandemic, but in fact that's what they are. People all over the world suffer from these often-debilitating conditions. They cripple otherwise-able men and women. They destroy lives, relationships, and companies. People do it on every level of their lives at almost every minute of the day, and it often leads to mental and physical disease and premature death.

If you're reading this, chances are either procrastination or overthinking (or both) are a problem in your life. So, I hope you don't feel alone, as it's a rare person who doesn't succumb to one or the other (or both). And the same things which inspire those unfortunate practices touch upon so many other facets of life that they cannot be ignored, or they will go on to spread like an infection. Anybody who procrastinates or overthinks has to get a grip on those practices now, there's literally no time to waste.

This book will provide you with everything you need to defeat those twin threats to your very life, those enemies of happiness and success. You will come to understand the sources of the emotions which inspire those behaviors. You'll have time-tested techniques which are clear and easy to understand and to put into practice to end and reverse the cycles which perpetuate procrastination and overthinking. And you'll learn to apply them to other facets of your personal and professional life to make your entire world a better and happier place. You'll master self-discipline, time management, relationships, all by finally coming to master your own inner self. It's well within your power, easier than you could have possibly imagined. All you need is the desire (which you've proven) and the commitment.

But don't let that word scare you off. It's a big part of conquering procrastination and overthinking, as it is a big part of anything you may pursue in life. If you've got the commitment, I've got all the information and applicable exercises you need.

And who am I? I'm Stewart Hunter, one of the proud and privileged writers here at Devon House Press. We are dedicated to sharing all the latest information to those in need of making their lives better. We believe everybody's life can be improved, and that this will elevate others and raise our entire society to a higher bar. We use the latest research technology and the latest research to give our readers the full breadth of understanding and all the tools they need to correct the often-deadly behavior in their lives. We remove the stumbling blocks to your success and happiness. And we're proud and pleased to do it.

Because we believe we're not just changing lives, we're *saving* lives. Not only will these techniques make you a better and happier individual, they will make you a happier partner in relationships, marriages, and families. Not only will they make you a better worker or manager, they will propel you up the ladder to greater successes. If you feel as if you're sliding down that ladder, the exercises in this book will reverse that trend! Not only will you learn things that will improve your health and wellbeing, you will learn things which just might prevent premature death.

I suffered from both procrastination and overthinking for most of my life. I always needed extensions on my tax returns, I was often late with credit card payments, and I paid the price in ruined credit and tax penalties. But I built my way back to a position of respect and considerable reward by using exactly these techniques. At the core of these practices is the *Pomodoro* technique, which we'll discuss in greater detail later in this book. But that system of breaking down one huge task into smaller milestones and using a schedule to keep the smaller milestones progressing toward the completion of the greater task, is key to the writing of this book itself! It's the way books are written, the way movies are produced, the way buildings, roadways, cars, and rockets are built. So, you're looking at proof-positive that these techniques work.

I got it in ahead of my deadline too.

Reading this book and coming to truly understand the concepts and practices cannot help but improve your life. If you take just one thing away from this book (improved self-efficacy, the *Eat the Frog* technique) and really apply it, your life will be improved, no question. Apply just two more (time logging, meditation) and your successes will accumulate faster than you can count them. And I'm certain you'll find that they all work together, that the success of one technique will inspire you to adapt yet another. They're all part of a tapestry of self-improvement techniques that will certainly enrich both your personal and professional life. You will learn to achieve any goal and reach your full potential, even to expand that potential! You'll learn to recognize the things that are holding you back and you'll have the tools to overcome them. You'll beat those life-crippling behaviors; procrastination and overthinking, but the benefits will go way beyond that. As I said, it stretches across the Earth and even beyond.

And it does. Read on and you'll see. Your whole world view is about to change for the better. Your life is on the precipice of great change. It's up to you!

But don't let procrastination separate you from these life-altering and life-saving techniques. Don't overthink it to a point where you make no decision at all. Don't let negative self-talk convince you that it won't work or that you're doomed to a life of failure. Those things have likely robbed you of your joy and success for too long. And it doesn't matter if you're a student, a teacher, or a retiree, you can still turn those negative behaviors around. You can still live your best life and be the best person you can be; better to yourself, better to your friends, better to your company, better to society. But you must do it now! There's a lot to cover and time is running out for us all. Let's face it, time is the one thing nobody can afford to waste.

And the particular problem here is that forestalling action is just the inspiration for the book, for my writing and you reading it. That means you'll have to conquer the very things which plague you in order to conquer the things that plague you. But as you'll quickly realize, it's just a matter of taking that first step to break that downward spiral. Just having this book open in front of you *is* that first step, you've already taken it! Now take the second step and read it.

What's more, this is information you can share with those you know and love. These practices are so widespread, and the remedies so logical and simple and effective, chances are you'll want to share this knowledge with your family and friends and coworkers alike. You might pass this information along to your boss or your superiors. They'll be impressed that you know these techniques and that you know how to use them, you're bound to do more than just make a good impression.

So, what are you waiting for? Just for me to end this introduction, I suppose, so that we can get on with the urgent business of changing your views of yourself and the world around you, improving both, and recreating your world as you never thought it could be. It's as simple as turning the page. So, let's get to it!

I

DIAGNOSING THE ROOT CAUSE

WHAT YOU SHOULD KNOW ABOUT PROCRASTINATION AND OVERTHINKING

YOU'RE NOT ALONE IN THIS

Procrastination is defined as postponing tasks, either knowingly or not. It's derived from the Latin *pro-crastinus*, meaning *belonging to tomorrow*. Of course, there's only so much anybody can accomplish in a day, and some things do have to be left to the next day. But when these things are habitually postponed, it's about more than just time management.

People procrastinate doing different types of things, and they do it all the time whether or not they realize it. Estimates are that roughly 20% of people surveyed consider themselves chronic procrastinators. Getting an extension to file tax returns is a classic example of simply putting off an unpleasant chore. Unfortunately, health care is often the subject of procrastination. But people also postpone plans to write a novel, take a vacation, and other pleasant pursuits.

Why is this? Are our daily lives so busy that we simply cannot make time, or are there other things at play? And though we can't add more hours to the day, we can recognize when we've fallen into a cycle of procrastination and how to get out of it, so that we're making the most of the hours and the days which we do have available to us. The old saying goes, "you only regret the things you didn't do." And the reason most people don't do these things is procrastination and over-thinking.

In our increasingly clamorous society, it's increasingly easy to procrastinate. The internet alone provides countless ways to waste time; from videos on YouTube to chatting with friends on Facebook or posting things to your Instagram or Twitter accounts. Countless cable and streaming channels provide more content than any person could watch in a lifetime. So, it's easy to put things off, altogether too easy.

What's important to remember is that virtually anything in life is more important than a video of a baby panda or a rerun of some TV show. Life is short, and procrastination only robs you of what little time you have. That's why it's so important to recognize this dangerous practice and to learn to control it. It's really quite easy, but it does require a bit of awareness and a clear head about what we're dealing with.

People have a variety of reasons for procrastinating and overthinking. They often set standards that are impossibly high, and therefore, they never try to rise to them. They may convince themselves that it's better not to take a risk and fail, or that everything in their lives should be easy and without challenge. When the challenge arises, the procrastinator my blanche at doing anything at all. Other insecurities, such as fear of personal rejection, may be factors as well.

To better understand what procrastination is, it's helpful to remember what it is not. Resting is not procrastination. Nobody can work non-stop; we all need to recharge our batteries. That's part of a well-balanced life. Similarly, procrastination is not laziness. Lazy people lack the goals or motivation to achieve at all. Procrastination happens when a person wants or needs to accomplish a goal but doesn't manage to get around to doing it. Often this is a question of motivation.

One way to look at procrastination is to examine the concept of motivation. If we're highly motivated, we're more likely to accomplish what we need to and less likely to postpone it. Fines and other criminal liability are great motivators to get those taxes filed, right?

But there are different types of motivation, and some are proved to be less successful than others. Extrinsic motivation, or a reward-based motivation, proves to stimulate less dopamine in the brain and therefore, result in a lesser performance. Goal-based motivation is stronger but may have a tendency to lose its potency after the goal is achieved. Intrinsic motivation has, at its core, an internal vision which carries over from goal to goal, one which expresses the creator's true goals in life. Some people used to say that pressure is a great motivator, but we know now that the stress it creates is almost always counterproductive.

Some people are negatively motivated to procrastinate, a sense of rebellion against having to do unpleasant chores in the first place.

However, one may fall into the habit of procrastination, recognizing the cycle is a good way to break it. Generally, procrastination begins with inaction, then guilt which leads to self-doubt, which leads to a feeling of helplessness. Basically, the protagonist may say of themselves, *"I didn't do it, I should have done it, maybe I can't do it, maybe I can't do anything."* Here we see the danger of overthinking, as mentally fixating on this cycle only makes the cycle stronger. More thinking along these lines only makes the problem worse.

Not a very pleasant or productive way to think, is it? Yet it's quite common and well within your ability to solve. One thing to keep in mind is that the cycle can be broken at any stage by simply doing the thing one didn't do in the first place.

A lot of people overcome procrastination by creating a personal vision, one which creates priorities that will motivate and sharpen focus not just one chore but every chore, as they all serve the overall personal vision in one way or another. To-do lists are also a popular and effective way to organize various chores and ensure they get done. Better habits reduce procrastination as well, and many people keep a habit list to help their development of new, better habits as they replace the old, more distracting habits. A lot of procrastinators set time aside for meetings with themselves, where they consider and reconsider their personal vision and to remain focused on their priorities.

THE CONSEQUENCES OF PROCRASTINATION AND OVERTHINKING

The results of procrastination and overthinking can be far-reaching and detrimental. It's about more than not getting some things done, it's about the long-lasting effects it can have on your life.

We've already considered the waste of time procrastination creates, years that pass unproductively, perhaps decades or even an entire lifetime. This causes shame, depression, and the downward spiral only gets worse. This creates life-changing opportunities to be missed, either because of depression, a feeling of helplessness to succeed, or simply lack of preparedness. Procrastination and overthinking are often at the root of all three. Procrastination can also prevent long-term goals from being achieved, as it stymies the sufferer who then cannot take the first crucial steps toward improving their lives and accomplishing their goals. Failure to achieve these goals can have career consequences, as a lack of training or development which prevents certain promotions. That lack of professional success can easily cause depression and decreased self-esteem. This can set the stage for poor decisions and lesser goals instead of smarter, long-term goals. This can be damaging to your reputation, further damaging career prospects, inspiring greater depression, and so on. As we can see, procrastination is a downward spiral.

The concrete examples of procrastination's corrosive effect on anybody's life are plain to see and wise to keep in mind. Procrastinating a visit to the doctor or dentist will almost certainly have adverse effects on your health. Procrastinate paying the utility bills and the utilities will be shut off. Miss the tax deadline and there will be fines and perhaps criminal persecution. Put off work or school assignments and you may be sanctioned with a demotion or a failing grade.

Studies also show that procrastinators are more likely to indulge in dangerous activities like smoking, taking controlled substances, unprotected sex, alcohol abuse, and poor driving habits.

At the same time, there can be some benefits to procrastination and overthinking. Taking a bit more time before doing a chore allows for reflection and consideration and may prevent a rushed and therefore lesser performance. Often, procrastination is really just prioritizing. You might do the easier chores on your to-do list first, putting off the more complex chore until the simpler ones are done. And oftentimes, procrastinating doesn't have any obvious long-term effects when the job does finally get done, even if it was at the last minute. A lot of procrastinators see it as a *no-harm/no foul* situation.

Let's take a closer look at overthinking on its own. If procrastination is the forestalling of a certain action, overthinking is often the cause. Examples of overthinking are quite commonplace, and it's an easy trap to fall into. You might be concentrating so hard on a work project that it keeps you up at night. Or you might be reliving an argument you had with a family member and be unable to get it out of your head. If so, you're probably overthinking.

Remember that thoughts cause emotions, and overthinking can create unwieldy, uncontrollable emotions.

Very often, anxiety is at the core of procrastination and overthinking. Anxiety is the normal reaction to stress, but ongoing anxiety is often a hazardous condition or set of conditions; generalized anxiety disorder, social anxiety, or panic disorder. Nearly 40 million American adults suffer from one type of anxiety disorder or another.

Overthinking can lead to analysis paralysis, wherein you may be spending so much effort considering different choices or scenarios that no initial choice is ever made, and nothing gets done at all.

Overanalyzing something can interfere with discovering the solution. Very often our focus can become so fixed on the problem that we lose sight of it. Taking a walk or taking a shower can sometimes break this cycle, as your focus is turned to something simple and mundane which takes little thought, and your mind is unlocked to re-examine the original problem. Overthinking often interrupts sleep patterns, which in turn can have a variety of detrimental effects on both your physical and mental health. Overthinking may trigger mental illnesses and even suicide!

There are a variety of ways you can combat overthinking, including being mindful of the moment and trying not to live too much in either the past or the future, and to be more forgiving of yourself. There are some things you can't control, after all.

And you're not alone. One University of Michigan study found that 52% of 45- to 55-year-olds overthink, and 73% of adults between the ages of 25 and 35 do as well.

A recent U.K. study showed that certain parts of the human brain are more creative when the cognitive process is quieted. According to the study, overthinking naturally thwarts with quieted, creative brain.

Overthinking also eats up a surprising amount of energy and can leave anyone exhausted and unable to break out of the procrastination cycle. And the stress of overthinking may produce the stress hormone called cortisol. But this hormone can be depleted, causing a sort of mental burnout.

Cortisol can also increase your appetite, which creates a pattern of stress eating. This may cause any number of detrimental conditions and diseases including obesity, diabetes, congestive heart failure, stroke, cancer, and any number of other life-threatening maladies. Weight gain can have psychological effects as well, creating depression, loss of self-esteem, isolation and loneliness, and these only contribute to the cycle of procrastination and overthinking.

A Harvard Medical school conducted a study on the brains of subjects at 60-70-years old and contrasted them to the brains of those 100 years old or even older. The results were that those who died earlier had less of the protein which quiets brain activity. Other studies indicate that this protein, RE1-Silencing Transcription (REST), may protect against Alzheimer's disease. But it can be depleted by overuse, which experts believe may be created, in these cases, by overthinking.

Cortisol and other hormones may elevate blood sugar levels and blood fats called triglycerides. That may lead to a host of maladies, including dizziness, fatigue, accelerated heartrate, headaches, difficulty swallowing, inability to concentrate, dry mouth, muscle tension, irritability, nausea, rapid breathing, nervous energy, twitching, trembling, and sweating.

If these hormones are not properly used by the body, the results may include digestive disorders, short-term memory loss, heart attack, premature coronary artery disease, muscle tension, and suppression of the immune system.

Meditation and exercise are good ways to combat overthinking, as is a worry log, or a diary of things which are worrisome or have to be dealt with, a kind of to-do list for your brain. Experts agree that the act of writing is a way to purge the subjects from your subconscious mind and stop the overthinking cycle. Therapy is often recommended, and a strong network of friends and family for support can often make all the difference.

PROCRASTINATION IS A CYCLE, IT EATS UP YOUR LIFE WITHOUT YOU KNOWING ABOUT IT

We've already taken a brief look at procrastination and overthinking as a cycle, feeding upon itself. Procrastination may begin with inaction which leads to guilt, which then may lead to self-doubt, resulting in a feeling of helplessness.

The cycle may also take on physiological aspects; poorer eating habits may create weight gain which adds to the depression, and that depression may trigger the overthinking which stimulates the brain hormones which motivate overeating.

But the cycle of procrastination and overthinking goes even deeper than that. Very often, procrastination begins with hopefulness and determination *("I'll start early this time")* which turns to pressure after the ensuing inaction *("I've got to get started!")*. Here's where anxiety and paralysis step in, and it only gets worse as the procrastinator enters false hope *("I can still do it!")* and then shame and self-recrimination *("Why can't I do this?")* and then often hopelessness *("I just can't do this!")* or a repeating of the cycle with renewed optimism *("I'll start early next time")*. The next day, it starts all over again.

To break this cycle, simply go to the second step. The first step is the same, hopefulness and determination *("I'll start early this time")*. But replace inaction with action in step two. Make a plan, put a to-do list together *("This is how I'll get this done")*. Then use a bit of discipline to avoid the pull of procrastination, *("Why am I resisting this?")* and then take action, even if it's only one step of the project *("I got this done")*.

Let's think of it another way: The various reasons people have for procrastinating, such as fear of failure or a presumption of ease in life, can be thought of as unhelpful rules or assumptions. Going into a task with such rules only creates disgust for the task, leading to distractions and other procrastination activities. They endure the consequences, such as stress or negative socialization, and then wind up procrastinating again the next time.

But a simple change in those unhelpful rules changes everything. Instead of a sense of entitlement, you might assume that most things worth doing in life are going to be a challenge, that nothing worthwhile is ever truly easy. Instead of fearing failure, tolerate the risk. Failure can be corrected, after all, and a failure to act is the true danger in these cases. Simply acting is a victory to a big degree. Changing those unhelpful rules into helpful rules changes the resulting emotion, which will be pride in the progress instead of disgust in the chore. This means dismissing the distracting, procrastination practices and completing the task at hand. The negative consequences of procrastination, the shame and self-doubt, are replaced by pride in achievement and new confidence to get such things done. That inspires you to get the job done the next time and not procrastinate at all.

Voila, the cycle is broken.

WHY IS IT SO IMPORTANT TO CRUSH OVERTHINKING AND PROCRASTINATION?

We've already taken a look at the consequences of procrastination and overthinking; the social pitfalls, the physical and mental and emotional toll it can take. But let's take a look at the other side of that coin and ask what the benefits come from *not* procrastinating or over-thinking.

In the same way that procrastinating and overthinking can severely limit what a person may accomplish over their lifetimes, it's also true that not procrastinating created a far more productive life. You may have no idea the things you're capable of or the successes which could be yours simply by making a few small changes to your outlook and your personal habits. The only way to fully plumb the depths of your potential is to act, and that means breaking the cycle of procrastination and overthinking.

Being more productive impacts more lives than just your own. You become an example to others to act and strive to achieve their own goals, and they go on to inspire others. That's a positive cycle you won't want to break, and it will go on endlessly if you remain productive.

You'll also manage to accomplish something; perhaps something small and private, like creating a piece of jewelry or perhaps something big and far-reaching, like creating a jewelry company.

One accomplishment will lead to another, opportunities create opportunities. But you'll only be able move onto the next project once you've completed the current one. Ergo, finish this and you can move on to the next. It'll be helpful if you don't overthink other projects too. Be in the moment and focus on what you're doing instead of what you did or didn't do in the past, or what you may or may not do in the future.

This way, you'll never find yourself in a mental rut, because your new goals and projects will keep you mentally and physically stimulated. And having more to do will encourage better time management.

Perhaps most importantly, you'll learn to take risks and conquer your fears. Franklin Delano Roosevelt famously said, *"The only thing we have to fear is fear itself,"* and it's a perfect way to think about procrastination and overthinking. Anxiety wells up and creates doubt and fear, preventing us from accomplishing the things we want and need to do. But quell the fear with a measure of acceptance, you'll find the courage to move ahead and do what needs to be done. Goals and dreams will come to life, and you will be free of the downward spirals of procrastination and overthinking.

But no book will solve this problem for you. This guide will help you take these steps on your own, create the life you really want. You see the need for a new and better outlook, and you're taking the first vital step on your journey to a happier life. But there's a way to go and little time to get there, so let's get to work and take a closer look at the effects of environment on procrastination and overthinking. That can make all the difference between wasting any more of your valuable time and achieving everything you've ever wanted to achieve.

YOUR ENVIRONMENT COULD BE DRASTICALLY AFFECTING YOUR PRODUCTIVITY LEVELS WITHOUT YOU REALIZING IT

YOU ARE SHAPED BY THE INFLUENCE OF THE PEOPLE AROUND YOU

The people, places, and things around you can have a powerful influence on you, just as you can have a powerful influence on them. It's worth noting here the difference between influence and control. Control is often a futile effort; so many chaotic things can happen throughout the course of a day, a week, or a month, that we can't possibly control all of it, no matter how hard we try. We often can't even control ourselves!

Influence, on the other hand, happens virtually effortlessly. We generally influence those closest to us more strongly than others, and we're likewise more greatly influenced by those who are closest to us. Think of parenting; children cannot always be controlled, but they are always influenced, and by their parents more than anyone else in the early stages of life. Similarly, a child cannot generally control their parents (this is not always true), although, they can influence them in any number of ways. Friends and peers become a major influence once we begin spending more time with them (in school and in the afternoons and weekends) than we spend with our parents (often restricted to a few hours during dinner, if that).

One of the crucial differences is that influence happens automatically, but control requires incredible effort.

So, in dealing with procrastination and overthinking, know first that the best you're likely to do is influence things, not control them; and in a lot of cases that's a lot easier and more effective.

But because influence happens without a concerted effort, one has to be careful not to inadvertently become a bad influence. This requires a little mental discipline, but it's well worth it for you and those around you.

Our moods can influence others, for example. If someone is riding high and another is feeling low, they're likely to draw each other toward a middle ground. Some people in their feelings, one way or the other, and tend to move less and move others more toward their own state of mind. This can be beneficial when the person is upbeat or positive, but when they're constantly negative the situation can be toxic for the other person.

Further complicating things, a single person may be stronger and more resilient on one day, less so on another. Holidays generally find some people on less-stable ground, for example. So, if you're one of them, and the holidays are coming around, it's wise to be aware of your tendencies so you can better control them. The same goes if you know somebody who endures this so you can avoid them during these vulnerable times.

When somebody is a constantly negative influence, there's little you can do to control their perspective. But you can influence by being a consistently better example and hope to elevate them to your level. This is often no easy task, as it means facing and overcoming your own personal negativity, something we can all be subject to from time to time. But that negativity is something to be conquered anyway, so this is as good a time as any!

Cleansing your psyche and elevating your positive influence is a good way to deal with negative influences, but it won't always be enough, and it takes a fair amount of time.

The effects of negativity, from within or without, can be dangerous and shouldn't simply be tolerated. Studies show that even small amounts of negative brain activity may weaken the immune system and lead to heart attack or stroke. According to Dr. Travis Bradberry, negativity can compromise the effectiveness of the neurons in the hippocampus, the part of the brain which handles memory and reasoning.

So, a lot of people recommend simply cutting such people out of your life. If you can't control or influence them, simply remove them from your environment. A principle of Nichiren Buddhism (the oneness of life and its environment) states roughly that our inner selves are reflected in our environment. When we change our environment, we influence our inner selves. If you cut those toxic people from your life, you cleanse your environment and thus, you cleanse your inner self.

Removing such people from your life will free you up to spend more time with better influences and create a stronger, more nurturing environment.

Find such positive influences in volunteer groups, which will elevate anybody's self-esteem. At work, mentors are always a positive influence despite the negative personalities you are likely to come across in almost any work environment.

If you can't avoid such people, set parameters. Physically distance if you can. A lot of negativity comes from self-pity. Instead of letting a complainer go on and on, ask them what positive steps they intend to take to correct their grievance. Resist engaging them in a debate over their feelings; you'll fail to influence them and only come off as bossy or argumentative. Nobody ever wins an argument.

Instead of asserting your perspectives or desires, which are basically irrelevant to such people, consider addressing them in a series of questions instead: *"How does that make you feel? What do you think you can do to change the circumstance so that you feel differently?"*

Again, consider setting the positivity bar higher, in ways that will influence your environment and yourself. Bring some snacks into work, pay somebody a compliment. That will elevate the positivity of everyone around you and that will help you maintain high positivity in return.

Researchers generally agree that negativity can be contagious. Research at the University of Indiana recently found that the negative opinions of others exert a stronger influence on others than positive opinions. Even those with positive opinions were more easily influenced by those with negative opinions, and discussion only increased the influence of the negative influence on the positive.

Psychologist Shilagh Mirgain, PhD puts it this way: "Happiness isn't just a personal experience, it is actually affected by the individuals around you." One person's negativity, for example, can radiate outward to others in that environment, affecting the entire group.

Mirgain's research also indicates that the happiness of a single individual may have a ripple effect of up to three degrees of separation (us, our friends, then our friends' friends). Mirgain also found that negative emotions have a greater impact than positive, often four to seven times greater.

To combat all this external negativity, consider sharing your feelings with those who are sympathetic (even to yourself if need be), surround yourself with positive people whenever possible, and get plenty of sleep. That'll help you to elevate your own positivity and, therefore, the positivity of the people around you.

All that negative energy can have a direct connection to both procrastination and overthinking. Because research increasingly indicates that procrastination isn't the result of poor time management, but of emotional conflict. In fact, poor time management is often seen as a symptom of an emotional problem, not the problem itself.

Rachel Eddins, a licensed professional counselor and American Counseling Association member, puts it this way: "There's not one answer to what procrastination is because [there are] so many things that lead to it." So, the best way to deal with procrastination is to first know what the main contributing factors are. Change those factors, change your environment, and you can change your mental state, better understand and overcome the tendency to procrastinate.

Procrastination is an avoidance strategy (literally), and those can create psychological pain which creates depression, anxiety, and other often debilitating conditions.

In 2007, University of Calgary psychologist Piers Steel described four causes of procrastination in what he calls the procrastination equation. The four causes should sound familiar by now:

Low Self-Efficacy: A person's confidence in being able to accomplish the task. Low self-efficacy contributes greatly to procrastination.

Low Value: The pleasantness of the task. Even boring or mildly painful tasks are lower value than extremely difficult tasks.

Impulsiveness: Ability to remain focused and resist distractions.

Delay: How much time until the task needs to be accomplished. The greater the delay, the more likely one is to put things off.

Steel combines these four elements into an equation which helps anybody calculate how likely they are to procrastinate, and it looks something like this:

Odds of Overcoming Procrastination = Self-Efficacy x Value / Impulsiveness x Delay

So, our self-confidence and the value of the task is divided by one's impulsiveness and the amount of delay. It's tricky, but it can help almost anyone figure out where they fall in the equation. Is self-efficacy the reason for your particular practice of procrastination? Increase it. Too impulsive? Decrease that according to the amount of delay you've got, and the equation should work out.

Here are some specific ways to deal with each of the four:

1. If self-efficacy is the cause, consider breaking the task down to smaller, more manageable blocks to create a series of small victories on your way to completion. That should boost your confidence and reassure you that you can get the job done.

2. If low value is the problem, find a way to increase the value. Make the boring task more pleasant by changing your environment, take your laptop to a public park or café and make it more of an enjoyable task, increasing its value.

3. If you're impulsive, remove those distractions. Turn off the internet, put your phone away, remove anything which distracts you. But don't feel badly about this, as research indicates that the human brain actually requires periodic distractions, it's programmed to work that way. Think about how a small animal will periodically check for danger in its

surroundings, no matter what the animal is doing; eating, drinking, cleaning itself. It's a survival impulse, and it's hardwired into the mammal brain.

4. If delay is your problem, create a series of mini deadlines, think of them as milestones. Time itself will help get the job done.

But outside the famous equation, there are other contributing factors to procrastination, and that brings us back to the environment. Because some procrastination is learned behavior, inherited from those closest to us and thus must likely to have the greatest influence on us. Perhaps a parent or boss or friend or coworker has the tendency, and this influence has affected your behavior too. You won't be able to do much for this person, but you can remind yourself that you can make your own decisions, and that not all influences are positive influences. Use some discipline to be a better influence on yourself.

Another word about controlling your environment before it controls you. The term *priming* refers to the concept of triggers. Walking past Starbucks may trigger your desire for a creamy, high calorie treat. Or walking past the gym may trigger your desire to work out and be healthier. And you can choose to walk past the gym instead of Starbucks if you change your route. Control the triggers in your environment and you can better control your triggers and the desires they inspire. This goes for smartphones, email notifications, and so on.

If you really want to defeat these little distractions, try temptation bundling. Instead of being low value tasks, consider how they relate to your long-term goals. That will make them high value tasks and they will be instantly be more enjoyable. Instead of dreading collecting your bank records for your accountant, think about how much money you'll save on your return this year. Instead of postponing mowing the lawn because of the drudgery of the task, think about how nice freshly cut grass smells, and how good your lawn will look

Rewarding yourself for little victories is another good way to keep yourself motivated. Did you collect and submit your bank records? Have a piece of cake! Mowed the lawn, did you? Sit back and enjoy the ball game! This series of rewards not only reinforces your sense of self-worth and accomplishment but it also gives you incentive to do the less-pleasant chores to begin with. It's what we call a win/win!

DON'T LET TOO MUCH PRESSURE DRAG YOU DOWN

Procrastination and overthinking, by you or someone you are close to, creates pressure. Lost time means harder work which needs to be done faster and, therefore, better. And while some people claim to work better under pressure, they're not taking into account the fact that there are different types of pressure stress. Athletes and artists may endure pressure stress, but this only helps them focus. The stress may even help the overall outcome. In this kind of stress, the person is fixed on the performance and that stress often creates transcendent results.

Destructive stress puts the focus on the person, not the task, and generally produces far lesser results. Destructive stress often results in mistakes. So, know what kind of pressure you're facing and which to avoid.

The pressure of procrastination and overthinking can come from inside and from outside. Other people's opinions, criticism, rejection, the external pressures often foster the tendency to overthink and procrastinate, as we've already discussed. Negative thinking around you can also be a real source of external pressure. But you can use that as motivation to do better, succeed, and be promoted to a better environment. The way you deal with overthinkers and procrastinators will determine how well you succeed. You can't control them, as we've seen, and even influencing them can be arduous. But if you can't avoid them, you'll have to deal with them somehow, something we'll discuss in greater detail in the next section of this book.

DISTRACTIONS AND TEMPTATIONS; IT WILL BE DIFFICULT TO DEFEAT THEM

And there's more to our environments than just the people inhabiting it. There are basically four different types of distractions; those you can control, those you cannot control, those which are annoying and those which are fun, but they all originate from our environment.

Some distractions are outside of your control, and they can be annoying (an office meeting) or fun (a dinner invitation). You can't prevent these, but you can be quick to return to work after either one with just a bit of self-discipline. Distractions which you can control can also be annoying (checking emails) or they can be fun (watching YouTube videos or posting on Twitter). Consider scheduling time for these distractions so they don't interfere with more important tasks. Set aside a few hours in the morning or evening for those distractions which you can control to make room for the distractions you can't control.

A study on distractions on focus included two groups; individuals who were promotion-focused and sought positive outcomes, and if individuals are prevention-focused, who tried to void negative outcomes. The study found that distractions, such as music, had little influence on the results. Rather, prevention-focused participants performed worse and enjoyed the task less than the promotion-focused test subjects.

But that doesn't mean distractions aren't still costly. You might spend one minute on your phone, but studies indicate that it may take over 23 minutes of wasted time to return to the task at hand.

Though distractions aren't always external. The left lateral prefrontal cortex of the brain may be impaired, making people more likely to succumb to the temptation of immediate satisfaction rather than long-term gain, which is just what a distraction often is.

LIVING WITH OVERTHINKERS AND PROCRASTINATORS

Often the problem of overthinking and procrastinating is part of the negative influence of others and your problem is having to deal with them. When you can't limit your exposure or try to redirect them in a positive direction, there are still good ways to deal with that negative influence, and to keep it from influencing you.

Don't minimize their perspective. Overthinkers are obsessing, that's true, but telling them that doesn't help. One might be moved to try to reduce the scope of the problem to relieve the overthinking, saying basically, "It's no big deal." But procrastination and overthinking are as much emotional problems as anything else, as we've seen. So, trying to approach it logically won't work, and it may even make fixation worse as the one who overthinks takes offense. Then they'll over-think *that* too.

Similarly, don't reduce the potency of their feelings. Somebody who's overthinking something can't just get over it. They're emotionally locked in, and just like telling them they have nothing to worry about, telling them they have no right to their legitimate feelings will only make things worse.

A lot of anxiety is irrational, so there's no point in asking somebody why they're overthinking things. Again, it's not about reason, it's about emotion. Try talking to them about the emotions they're processing instead of the thoughts they're processing.

It also doesn't help to compare the overthinker's dilemma to anybody else's. These challenges are different for everybody and they don't all handle them in the same way. Nobody else's dilemma is going to be of very much use.

Strangely, overthinkers aren't often looking for solutions or recom-mendations, much as they would seem to be seeking that very thing. Because it's not about reason but emotion, overthinking and fixating on a thing is often a matter of emotional release. Sometimes, a person just wants to vent. They're more fixated on the problem than the solution. It may seem irrational, and it very often is. But overthinking and procrastination are emotion-based, after all.

In the same way, reassurance can be of little value to the overthinker. They're not thinking as much as they are feeling, remember that.

Overthinkers don't overthink everything, just some things. If you know a particular overthinker, reflect on the pattern of what they're talking about consistently. That will direct you in how to answer them.

Emotions tend to fester for the overthinker, which only makes sense. Very often, they're looking for a way to process all that emotion. But as a result of all that emotion and confusion, overthinkers are often exhausted, nervous, and agitated. Keep that in mind when dealing with them or avoiding them entirely.

But for now, let's take a closer look within to see what you can do to improve your own productivity and peace of mind.

STOP THE SELF-SABOTAGE! YOU, YOURSELF, ARE THE PROBLEM

S elf-sabotage, or the practice of either actively or passively preventing one's own success, can take a variety of forms. It can be active, such as substance abuse. It can be passive, such as with procrastination. But it's often dangerous and can be devastating.

Interestingly, the same things which motivate people to procrastinate also motivate self-sabotaging behavior in general; a lack of self-worth, a fear of success and failure, a desire for control.

Self-sabotaging is often indicated by the same red flags which indicate procrastination and overthinking; Prioritizing instant gratification over long-term benefits, avoiding necessary tasks, not prioritizing self, focusing on self-defeating thoughts.

And the same techniques you may use for procrastination and over-thinking are comparable to the techniques you'd use to deal with all the self-sabotaging behaviors; positive thinking, achievable goals to bolster self-efficacy, adjusting environment to limit distractions and negative influences.

YOUR HEAD IS FILLED WITH A LOT OF THOUGHTS, AND IT'S NOT HELPING YOU ONE BIT

Our days are filled with all manner of distractions and things which require our attention. This certainly doesn't do any good for those who tend to overthink or procrastinate. And all that clutter in our environment surely infiltrates our psyches. Remember that our environments mirror our psychological states.

But what kind of thoughts are streaming around in our brains, and how do we control them? The first step is to identify one type of thought from another and deal with each in the appropriate fashion.

There are basically three different kinds of thoughts: Necessary thoughts relate to your daily routine ("What am I going to have for dinner?" or "What's my website password?"), while waste thoughts - waste thoughts have no constructive use at all ("What if this happens?" "Why did that person say such a thing to me?") These are often related to past or future events, not events in the current moment, and concentrating on the past or the future instead of the present is a big part of both procrastination and overthinking.

Then there are negative thoughts, which are harmful to you and to others. Perhaps not surprisingly, negative thoughts are primarily centered on five common vices; anger, lust, greed, ego, and attachment.

The human brain exhibits signs of a negativity bias, the tendency to focus on negative thoughts. This was a survival tactic for our ancient ancestors, but in the modern era it's often a source of anxiety and depression.

Negative thoughts are generally inspired by unsatisfied expectations in disagreements, in laziness, racism, criticism, jealousy, hate, and an excess of power. They're born of bitterness, frustration, and dissatisfaction.

Positive thoughts, on the other hand, redirect our attention away from those common vices and toward the virtues of prioritizing love, peace, purity, joy, and power. These are the thoughts which drive our better selves and inspire our greatest accomplishments.

But of all the different kinds of thoughts, positive thoughts can be the most challenging to pursue, as they require a tolerance for discomfort, facing problems and low value tasks, and considerable self-discipline and inner peace. A person must be mindful of these challenges and reward themselves with praise for the small accomplishments, reassuring one's own psyche of self-efficacy and of the high value of sometimes-unpleasant tasks. It's a matter of will to a large extent, but that doesn't make it as miserable as it sounds. Remember to congratulate yourself for the little wins, remember how the little tasks add up to great accomplishments, that's not so hard.

Or consider thoughts as being in three classes. Insightful thoughts are used for problem solving, experiential thoughts focus on a task at hand, and incessant thoughts are the kind of chatter which distract us and cause us to overthink events in the past or the future.

Doctor Albert Ellis created an A-B-C approach to defeating incessant thinking. According to Dr. Martin Seligman, considered the father of positive psychology, a negative thought loop has three components; adversity, beliefs, and consequences. An unfavorable event creates adversity, which inspire narratives that become our beliefs. Those beliefs influence our actions, and those actions have natural consequences.

But you can add a fourth component, disputation, wherein you dispute the beliefs and correct them before they lead to their natural consequences. In other words, you can always talk yourself down from the pitch of your negative beliefs.

Your adversity, for example, might be in filing your taxes. There's a lot of miserable paperwork involved, even if you hire an accountant. You may tell yourself it's just too much to deal with, a narrative, and then believe that narrative. But you can dispute that belief at any time in the cycle simply by reassuring yourself that you can collect the documents and that your taxes will be filed on time. Believe it and do it and then *that* becomes the narrative.

Another way to disrupt incessant thinking is to replace it with a different type of thought; try experiential thinking instead, or insightful thinking.

Knowing what kind of thoughts you're having will help you to better control them and resist being controlled by them.

Bloom's taxonomy lists six types of thinking skills ranked simple to complex: Knowledge (remembering and recalling), comprehension (interpreting meaning and understanding), application (using old information in new situations), analysis (categorizing, differentiating, and examining), synthesis (combining different applications as necessary), and evaluation (critical analysis).

Negative thoughts can also be influenced by cultural (how a group expresses itself), genetic (how a family expresses itself), and physical considerations (how an individual express themselves). Racism may be an example of cultural negative thoughts, for example; a family feud may be a genetic negative thought, and a mental impairment such as bi-polar disorder may be creating negative thoughts born of a physical consideration.

But there are ways to counter these negative thoughts. Changing an external situation (such as divorcing an abusive spouse), shifting attention (to focus on the positive instead of the negative in a given situation) or re-appraising a situation (to see the benefit instead of the drawback of a certain event).

Researchers have found that genetics determine 50% of happiness, circumstances such as wealth and health accounts for 10%, Shifting or re-appraising, the internal and intentional efforts to achieve happiness, account for the other 40%.

There's also the cognitive triangle, which holds that our mental state relies upon the interworking of three major components of our psyche; feelings, thoughts, and behaviors. Each influences the other, and a sound footing for each is required for a balanced mental and physical state.

You may think you're hungry for a delicious but unhealthy cheeseburger because you deserve it, and that may encourage you to feel that you need it from sheer hunger, and your behavior is going to be to eat that cheeseburger. So, use a bit of mental discipline and replace the unhealthy cheeseburger with a yummy veggie-burger and let your feelings and thoughts continue as they are.

One great way to combat negative thoughts is to be aware of them and to employ *cognitive decentering*, which means you see a troubling event as just that, an event, and not a reflection of the self. Events are often independent of the self, as they happen externally and not internally. The key is to not internalize them and let them remain external.

DIAGNOSING YOURSELF: ARE YOU A PROCRASTINATOR? IF SO, WHICH TYPE?

As we have seen, procrastination is one of the classic methods of self-sabotage. But not all delays of performance are procrastination, only the chronic, habitual delaying of tasks. But we've also seen that there are different ways to procrastinate, different reasons for doing so, and so there are different ways of interrupting the procrastination cycle.

But let's take a closer look at different ways a person may procrastinate, and this comes down to personality types. Different people may form different procrastination personalities, if you will. For example:

Some procrastinators may be described as *perpetual lovers*. This people-pleaser may be stuck in a place of inaction for fear of hurting others or of being judged by them. We've already noted that fear of rejection is a big part of procrastination, after all. This person worries about how they're perceived, they seek not to be disruptive, they fear to be unloved or unwanted.

Some procrastinators are more like *error officers*. This is the perfectionist procrastinator who'd rather do nothing that do the wrong thing.

A *small player* protagonist is timid, afraid of the adverse effects of change, and procrastinating makes that possible. A *hidden gem* or *imposter* procrastinator may be insecure (such as a teenage girl or an incompetent worker or a liar) and a *poor thinker* procrastinator may be confused about social norms (a wealthy Christian perhaps). A procrastinator may also be a dreamer and not a doer.

Now that you know who you are and why you're procrastinating, let's move on to something everybody has, and nobody wants ... bad habits.

YOU'VE DEVELOPED BAD HABITS THAT YOU CAN'T GET RID OF?

Self-sabotage is basically a collection of bad habits; substance abuse, overthinking, procrastination, inaction. All comprise different sets of bad habits. If you overthink or procrastinate, the chances are good that you've developed some bad habits. And the fact that you're reading this book means that you want to get rid of them

So, let's get to it.

Some bad habits are very common to procrastinators of all types, so look out for these red flags.

Addictive habits like eating, drinking, or drug use has an immediate calming effect, but only contributes to procrastination. Procrastinators envy hard workers, and for good reason. They're also chronically unreliable, even for themselves.

Lack of physical fitness and weight gain are symptomatic of the procrastinator's lifestyle, as stress eating and no time to exercise prove a one-two punch to the body's chemistry.

You're always in a hurry because you're leaving things to the last minute, creating a constant rush to get them done. You only clean when you have an even more boring task to do. You may be easily stressed. You may stress clean only when a more stressful task needs to be done.

Too much social media is a big red flag.

Weekdays and weekends blur into each other, since you're spending your weekends finishing the tasks you postponed from the work week. But weekends are important for preventing burnout.

Oversleeping; it's a classic delaying tactic, even if you don't realize it … because you're asleep.

How many times has your boss called you up for being late and you were sleeping? You know better.

You round up to the hour to forestall a task even for a few precious minutes. Instead of starting a task at 7:52, you'll wait until 8:00. At 8:05, you'll wait until 9:00.

You may be collecting smartphone apps, classic distraction devices.

You may be giving advice which you yourself don't follow. Why not? You've mastered through research that which you don't really know in practice. And that brings us to the Dunning-Kruger Effect.

Here's a helpful exercise: Make two lists; one of the numbers of your uncompleted plans and another list of episodes of your favorite TV show. If the first is longer, you know you're procrastinating.

Before we move onto the Dunning Kruger effect, let's talk about quitting bad habits. Habits easy to pick up but hard to quit are smoking and drinking. There are a number of reasons for this; some chemical and some psychological.

When you want to give up a habit, consider taking up the opposite habit. Instead of quitting smoking, take up the habit of becoming a nonsmoker. Replace that habit with another; walking, juggling, anything.

THE DUNNING-KRUGER EFFECT

Perhaps you've heard the old saying, "The more we learn, the less we know." It's about how humility comes with wisdom. Mathematician and Nobel laureate Bertrand Russell put it this way: "The fundamental cause of the trouble in the modern world today is that the stupid are cocksure while the intelligent are full of doubt."

So, researchers David Dunning and Justin Kruger set out to do an experiment on the certainty of one's own opinion and how it correlates to their actual ability. What they found was that certainty about a certain fact or circumstance was at its peak when the test subject was at the minimal level of competence. Increased competence created a lower level of certainty at first, but that rose with increased competence. The more we learn, the less we know.

The reason for this is a tendency to overestimate one's ability. Only education and wisdom can correct this overestimation. Many believe that those who are competent expect competence in others and therefore, estimate their own abilities as merely average. The less competent likewise expect others to be equally incompetent, and they can therefore assume that they are superior in their knowledge or capacity.

Furthermore, the study proved that the competent, when given an opportunity to self-assess, had no awareness of their incompetence. So not only do the incompetent overestimate their own abilities, they are impervious to any argument to the contrary. You cannot explain to an incompetent person their own incompetence. Largely it's a failing of logic. They cannot adequately use logic, as they are incompetent, therefore they cannot understand or accept it.

So, the first thing to do is make sure you yourself are not suffering from this widespread effect. Are you humble enough to know that you could be wrong, or that you might be acting from an emotional instead of rational place? How certain of your position are you? The more certain you are, the weaker ground you may be standing on.

And in dealing with others, if you can recognize the Dunning-Kruger effect, you'll know how to deal with those who are exhibiting it. Don't try to reason, as this person is not coming from a rational position. You may try to educate them, as increased knowledge is the only way to combat ignorant confidence, but don't expect them to digest your facts and be informed. They won't be moved by facts or logic because their position is not based on either one and their ability to see that is close to nil.

ARE YOU ARE OVERTHINKING IT? DO YOU KNOW WHY?

Overthinking comes in two forms; ruminating about the past and worrying about the future. Overthinking has its own set of bad habits too, so the better you recognize them the more quickly you can reverse them.

If you're an overthinker, you can't stop worrying or worry about things you can't control. You constantly reflect on your mistakes and relive unpleasant moments over and over in your mind.

Overthinkers tend to ask "what if..." questions endlessly and have difficulty sleeping because their brains won't stop circling around these negative thoughts.

You replay conversations in your head, regretting things you didn't say. You spend a lot of free time thinking about the hidden meaning behind things people say or events that occur.

You dwell on it when someone says something or behaves in a manner you don't like. You may also hold grudges and begin to feel paranoid that others are actively working against you. You spend so much time either dwelling on past events or worrying about the future that I often miss what's going on in the present.

Overthinkers are often overconfident in their own opinions and fixate on the opinions of others and are often pessimistic about what those thoughts are.

Overthinkers also fixate on what the deeper meaning behind some events might be, even when there might not be any deeper meaning or personal significance there. Overthinkers tend to want strict control over thoughts and actions and have little tolerance for spontaneity.

Some helpful ways to defeat overthinking can be used for other habitual patterns as well, including knowing and avoiding your triggers, be aware when you're doing it, and be aware of how essentially useless overthinking is. A forced distraction is another handy way to derail overthinking. Just apply your attention to something else … anything else.

Since overthinking focuses either on the past or the future, focus instead on the present. Meditation can help, as we've already discussed.

A GOOD NIGHT'S SLEEP OR ONLY A FEW HOURS? EITHER WAY, IT WILL AFFECT YOUR DAY

Not getting enough sleep is a common form of self-sabotage and very common to procrastinators and overthinkers alike. It's often the result of spending long, last-minute hours completing unfinished tasks, or from tossing and turning while overthinking one event or another. But it's very detrimental to your mental and physical health and only furthers any downward spiral.

Most adults require between seven and nine hours per night, teenagers and children a bit more as they expend so much more energy during the day. While distractions like TV and video and the internet can rob us of our sleep, good diet and exercise can contribute to a healthy sleep cycle.

A healthy sleep cycle has been proven to have beneficial effects on metabolism, mental wellbeing, sex drive, and fertility.

On the other hand, sleep deprivation is known to make people vulnerable to reduced cognition, attention lapses, mood shifts, and delayed reactions. It is also connected to type 2 diabetes, obesity, heart disease, high blood pressure, stroke, overall poor mental health, and premature death. Sleep deprivation is also associated with impulsive behavior, anxiety, paranoia, depression, bipolar disorder, and suicide. Signs and symptoms include excessive sleepiness, frequent yawning, daytime fatigue, and irritability. Sleep deprivation may also weaken your immune system.

The digestive system is also vulnerable to damage from too little sleep.

Sleep affects the levels of the hormones ghrelin and leptin, which control the body's feelings of fullness and hunger. Leptin is an appetite suppressant and ghrelin is the body's natural appetite stimulant. Too little sleep reduces leptin and increases amounts of ghrelin. The result is midnight snacking, overeating, weight gain, and the resulting heath issues.

Sleep deprivation also reduces the amount of insulin, which helps to reduce blood sugar levels, released by your body after meals. It is also associated with decreased hormone production, such as testosterone.

The human body has an internal body clock which regulates the sleep cycle. The 24-hour cycle is called the *circadian rhythm.* The rhythm includes a sleep drive which gets stronger as the cycle works through. That sleep drive, called *homeostasis,* may have links to an organic compound produced in the brain called *adenosine.* Adenosine increases throughout the day and are broken down during sleep.

Light also plays a big part in the circadian rhythm. The brain's hypothalamus has a cluster of cells known as the *suprachiasmatic nucleus.* These cells process signals from the eyes to the brain during exposure to natural light. This is what tells the brain if it's day or night.

With the loss of natural light, the body releases the hormone melatonin, which induces sleep. Natural morning light stimulates the body to create the hormone cortisol, which we've already taken a look at. Cortisol promotes alertness and energy.

So, if your sleeping habits are irregular, consider the effect of light in the room, too much or too little. Improve your diet and exercise regimen and get at least eight hours sleep a night.

But there are a variety of tips and tricks to help ensure a good night's rest. You may consider establishing a realistic bedtime and do not vary. Go to bed at the same time every night, and at a reasonable time too. This will establish a healthy and consistent sleeping pattern.

Temperature and light have a big effect on sleeping patterns, so keep the lights low and the temperature reasonable. Some people disallow TVs, computers, and smartphones in their bedrooms to prevent distractions and unnatural light.

Since the body has to work to digest food and drink, a lot of experts recommend staying away from alcohol, caffeine, or large meals in the few hours before bed. Abstain from caffeine, alcohol, and large meals in the hours leading up to bedtime. Experts recommend avoiding tobacco at night, as nicotine is a stimulant.

Daytime exercise is good for expending extra energy and readying the body for a sound sleep. Taking a hot bath or meditating before bed can be good strategies for a better night's sleep.

Some people in our frenzied modern world don't have that luxury. Some may be shift workers, for example, and must wake and sleep contrary to the cycle of morning and night. These folks can still take measures, including naps, limiting shift changes, and maintaining healthy lighting.

The flipside of sleep deprivation is too much sleep, and that can be detrimental as well.

Hypersomnia is a medical disorder causing sufferers to sleep for extended periods at night and remain tired throughout the day. The condition causes people to suffer from extreme sleepiness throughout the day, which is not usually relieved by napping. Hypersomnia is associated with memory problems, low energy, and anxiety.

Depression, alcohol abuse, and some pharmaceuticals can lead to oversleeping as well.

Oversleeping can lead to a number of dangerous conditions.

Oversleeping can contribute to obesity. According to a recent study, people who slept nine hours or more per night were over 20% more likely to become obese over a period of six-years than test subjects who slept the standard seven or eight hours.

Oversleeping has a certain effect on neurotransmitters in the brain, including serotonin. This may cause people who are prone to headaches to suffer from them as a result of too much sleep.

Fifteen percent of people with depression sleep too much, and those irregular sleeping habits may only contribute to the problem.

One study showed that women who slept between 9 and 11 hours were almost 40% more prone to heart disease than women who slept the standard eight hours per night. Inflammation is also found to be more common in those who oversleep.

Diet can have a strong connection to oversleeping. If you oversleep, consider changing your diet to increase amounts of these important nutrients which you may be lacking: Theobromine, which is found in chocolate; dodecanoic acid, which is found in coconut and palm kernel oil; Choline, found in fish, shrimp, turkey, soy, eggs, and some leafy greens; selenium, common to fish, turkey, shrimp, beef, chicken, brazil nuts, and some whole grains; lycopene is found in watermelon, red cabbage, cooked tomatoes, red peppers, and guava; phosphorus can be found in eggs, sunflower seeds, lean meats, lentils, tofu, fish, and pumpkin and sunflower seeds.

Sleep is crucial to a healthy happy life, and either too little or too much can both cause life-threatening problems and be symptomatic of them as well. But sleep patterns can be improved in a few basic and easy-to-manage ways. And once you're more alert and well-rested, you'll be able to deal with the fears that are derailing your best efforts during your waking *and* sleeping hours.

THE FEAR INSIDE THAT YOU DON'T EVEN REALIZE THAT EXISTS

We've already taken a look at analysis paralysis, or what happens when a person is so beguiled by their choices that they make no choice at all. Largely, this is founded in the fear of making the wrong choice. Fear is at the heart of a lot of conditions like this one, and it's an emotion that's well worth understanding.

FAILURE, EVERYONE FEARS IT, BUT SHOULD YOU?

Nobody sets out to fail. But it happens, even despite our best efforts or intentions. George Washington and Abraham Lincoln faced failure after failure on their way to the crucial successes which ensured the survival of their country. Everybody faces failure in big ways and little; missing a job promotion, getting a bad report from the doctor, missing a green light or missing a deadline. So, failure is something we're essentially programed to accept.

What we really fear, however, is the shame associated with fear; the anger of others who may be disappointed, the resultant rejection which may occur as a result of that failure. It's the shame that gets us.

Unlike guilt, which makes us feel bad about our actions, or regret, which makes us feel bad about our efforts, shame is about who we are. It addresses the issue of self-efficacy which is at the heart of procrastination and overthinking. Our egos and self-esteem may feel threatened by shame in particular.

Overly critical adults often cause children to internalize these damaging mindsets. Fear-based rules and ultimatum cause many children to ask for reassurance and permission, and this need for validation often carries into adulthood.

Fear of failing can often inspire insecurities and uncertainties about what other people's impressions or interests are, what future possibilities may be or be limited to, makes you worry about what other people think about you. It addresses issues of self-confidence and encourages a general lowering of the bar in order to prevent the risk of trying and failing at something truly challenging and which would be thusly rewarding.

Failure tends to lead to overthinking as well, locking a person in a cycle of imagining a different outcome based on other things which could have been said or done. Fear of failure (or shame, as you like) can manifest itself in the physical, creating last-minute headaches, stomach aches, sweating, fever, and other things which may prevent action and thus the possibility of failure. Distractions and excuses for running out of time are two other classic symptoms of fear of failure.

One good way to deal with all this is to simply own it. Accept that failure and shame are the risk that anybody takes when they try to achieve something. Know the difference between failure and shame; accept the failure and reject the shame. There is an old adage my own father often shared with me: *"Always do your best. It's all that you can do, and all anybody can ask of you."* So, if you did your best and failed, what reason for shame should there be in failure? Failure is a steppingstone to success, after all. Another adage, popular among artists, goes: *"If you never fail, you're not really trying."* So, go ahead and fail and don't be ashamed. The real shame comes from not trying at all.

Oddly, it's often the most successful people who have a fear of failure, as their identity is so closely related to their success. For them, failure is the antithesis of life. It can boggle artists as well, creating mental blocks which prevent the very creativity they need to succeed.

While those mental blocks can be debilitating, others needn't be. There are things in life you cannot control, there are things which you can control. Focus on them. If your goal is to get a new job but you don't know the right people, focus on meeting the right people!

We've all heard of phobias, irrational and debilitating fears. Heights, snakes, enclosed spaces and wide-open spaces all their associated phobias. So too is there a phobia of failure; atychiphobia.

Atychiphobia is more than just a trepidation about failure or a concern about what others may think or even overthinking about what could be or could've been. It's a paralyzing fear which can over-take your body or mind. Physical symptoms of such phobias include quickened heart rate, difficulty breathing, tightness or pain in the chest, dizziness or lightheadedness, hot or cold flashing, digestive problems, trembling or shaking, or sweating. Emotional symptoms include intense anxiety or panic or anxiety, an overwhelming flight impulse, a loss of control and detachment from one's self, fear of powerlessness, or death.

Previous failures or a learned fear of failure can contribute to devel-oping a case of atychiphobia. The phobia can also be a learned or inherited condition if passed on by a parent or friend in a process called *observational learning experience.* Even just reading or hearing about it may trigger informational learning and encourage manifestation of the phobia (or any phobia).

WE ALL KNOW ABOUT THE FEAR OF FAILURE, BUT DO YOU HAVE A FEAR OF SUCCESS?

It's almost a cliché, and one that's hard to digest. Who's afraid of being wealthy and successful? Well, it's like the fear of failure, which is more about shame. The fear of success is more about fear of change.

Introverts tend to have a fear of success, as they shy away from the extra attention success brings. Success can breed contempt and cost a person friendships. Success can be both fleeting and corrupting and is rarely all that it's cracked up to be. This is a kind of *backlash avoid-ance* which is behind a lot of cases of fear of success. It's about a fear of change and what that change might bring.

One may also fear that they don't deserve the success, and that they'll be revealed as an imposter and humiliated.

Signs of a fear of success include low goals, procrastination, perfectionism, quitting, self-destructive behavior, which should now be quite familiar to the reader. Ways to combat it should be just as familiar.

Explore the origins of the fear, the type of fear, the reasons for it. Own it and understand it. Exercising, dieting, having a sound sleep cycle, socializing, even journaling can help. Some recommend visualizing success, some using image boards to compile pictures of the things they wish to accumulate.

If you're having what is sometimes called a *panic attack*, there are ways to bring yourself back down to Earth. Take a walk, do some breathing exercises, call a friend for some support.

Journaling his highly recommended for the fear of success. It's recommended to take a half hour or so in the day, preferably at the same time every day, to write down whatever thoughts you may have on the fear of success; memories of the past, problems in the present, or plans for the future.

Fear of success, like all phobias, is an avoidance strategy. If you're afraid of rats, you'll avoid them. Avoiding praise or opportunities or even romances is how the fear of success may manifest itself.

The fear of success can actually take on familiar shapes, six different archetypes of the fear of success. Knowing which one mirrors your

own feelings and understanding that archetype will help you overcome it and your fear of success.

- The *Goal Addict Type 1* is the overachiever. The goal addict
  is set on his or her goals high and proud of those
  achievements. For the Goal Addict type 1, failure is
  untenable but always likely.
- The *Goal Addict Type 2* is the other side of the goal addict
  coin; they set the bar low and succeed at that. For them, the
  risk of failure is fairly low.
- The *Disbeliever* is skeptical of success, that it can be
  achieved by him or her or by anyone else. For the
  Disbeliever, the risk of failure is almost nil, and any failure
  will be blamed on someone or something other than his or
  herself.
- The *Saboteur* is the counterpart to the Disbeliever. The
  Saboteur is, like the Disbeliever, a fatalist, but he goes into an
  essentially doomed effort with a positive, not a negative
  attitude. For the Saboteur, failure if virtually certain.
- *Half-Hearters* are somewhere between the Disbeliever and
  the Saboteur. The Half-Hearters will play along but
  contribute nothing, offer the unspoken skepticism of the
  Disbeliever and a counterfeit version of the Saboteur's
  willingness to participate.
- *Inventors* are centered on their own efforts but may resist
  being part of a bigger team effort. This sense of introversion
  works against their efforts to succeed.

NOTHING LESS THAN PERFECT KEEPS YOU POSTPONING YOUR DECISIONS AND ACTIONS

You hear it a lot these days: "Don't let the perfect be the enemy of the good." And it's as true for procrastination and overthinking as for anything else. Perfectionism is the enemy of the protagonist, for sure. We've already looked at how perfectionism works against the protagonist's best efforts to break the cycle and get things done in a timely fashion. What the perfectionist protagonist often forgets is that nothing is ever perfect, good is often good enough. What matters is that the task is accomplished to the best of the performer's ability, after all. That's always better than having the task not be completed at all.

How do you know if you're actually a perfectionist, and not just trying very hard? Perfectionists focus too much on the results and too little on the process. It doesn't matter how it gets done, as long as the results are up to par. Every achievement fades behind the next one. No victory is good enough, the work is never done. One project must follow the next, and none are ever really good enough. The perfectionist also beats himself or herself up over the results, any results; they're never good enough. The perfectionist is also a fast worker, not stopping until a job is done.

They sound like admirable traits, but they can cause a lot of procrastination and overthinking, among other destructive behaviors. The problem is that the procrastination is born of misguided activity, which is different than inactivity. The procrastinator may believe he or she is hard at work, but the task is not being accomplished for all the preparation being done instead.

And the higher the stakes, the greater the risk, the greater chance for failure and therefore, procrastination.

To combat the effects of perfectionism, one only has to reassure themselves that a thing doesn't have to be perfect, simply lower the par on the process and the results. Don't let the perfect be the enemy of the good.

Use design thinking to emphasize the process over the result. If the process is sound, after all, the result should be too. Give yourself time to be unproductive to rest your creative, physical, and mental resources.

Consider an action-anxiety rubric. In two columns, list a series of tasks, or actions, and the associated anxiety you may have with finishing those tasks. Pick the smallest one and resolve it. That will bolster your confidence and help break down the cycle of procrastination.

Stanford University psychologist Carol S. Dwick, Ph.D., believed that people generally had either one of two mindsets, fixed or growth. A fixed mindset focuses on current talents or skills or intelligence, believing that they are fixed in stone and cannot be developed. These people may believe, for example, that musical talent must be innate and cannot truly be learned. A growth mindset holds the opposite set of beliefs, that a set of skills or the breadth of intelligence can be expanded and improved. For this mindset, almost anybody may develop skills to become a musician or essentially anything else.

The fixed mindset tends to hinder growth and evolution, while the growth mindset has the opposite effect, encouraging growth and development.

We've looked at the basic causes of procrastination and overthinking and investigated the damaging effects and ways of coping. So, let's move onto Section 2 of this book and develop more specific solutions to break the cycle and eradicate the problems of procrastination and overthinking from your life forever!

II

DEVELOPING THE EXACT SOLUTIONS TO FIX THE PROBLEM

STOP YOUR PROCRASTINATING!

BE HONEST, HOW MUCH DID YOU PROCRASTINATE TODAY?

To be fair, you may not even realize you're procrastinating at all, never mind about how much. But a recent study indicates that only 18% of procrastination can be attributed to simple task aversion. So, what's going on with the other 82%?

Here we return to illusion of productivity. We may think we're busy, but we busy ourselves with tasks other than the one which needs to get finished. We're so busy preparing, we neglect to perform. But there are other, unconscious ways we procrastinate every day without even knowing it!

Blaming others is one way of procrastinating. Since so many of our daily tasks are reliant upon others also doing their part, it's altogether too easy for anyone to simply blame the performance of their counter-part. It is a passive/aggressive move, but very common with procras-tinators.

We've already looked at how perfectionism can cause analysis paraly-sis, but this is also one of the unconscious ways of procrastinating. The perfectionist feels that they're moving slowly and surely, but often they're not moving forward at all. Worry, depression, fear of failure, and overthinking are common to the perfectionist protagonist.

Sometimes procrastination isn't related to the act at all, but the moti-vation; not the what but the why. Take marriage, for example. People have reasons (why) for getting married (what). They've committed to both, so they no longer question *why* they got married ... only *how* to stay married!

But procrastinators often can't answer the reason why, so they waffle. This could be why a lot of people put off the decision to get married. Under analysis, they can't answer the question of why they should do it, so they don't. This is increasingly common among millennials, among whom marriage rates have fallen drastically.

On the other hand, studies show that committed action produces more positive results.

As an exercise, imagine yourself in two months, and then imagine yourself in ten years. How will your choices affect you in two months or in ten years? Keep the long-term consequences in mind. Be aware of the subconscious ways you might be sabotaging yourself with procrastination and you'll be able to tackle them consciously.

One good way of dealing with unconscious procrastination is to keep a time log. For an entire month, write down everything you do and when you do it, in half-hour blocks if you can. At the end of the month, review the log and you'll see where and when you were less productive, even if you didn't realize it at the time. It will also illustrate why you were unproductive. You're bound to see patterns in time and activities.

When doing your time log, consider categorizing time spent for different functions. For example, you may spend your time doing paid work (your job), passion work (a side project), professional development (networking or job seeking), personal development (journaling or taking classes), relationships (friends, family, dating), play (shopping, surfing the internet or watching TV), wellness (exercise and self-care), support work (mentoring, volunteering), distractions (daydreaming) and maintenance (daily chores). Almost everything you do will fit into one of these categories. Your time log will help you identify how you're spending too much, or too little, of your time.

There'll be crossover, of course. Cooking may be classified as maintenance, but if you enjoy it, it can also be passion work, fun, or personal development. But when you're doing your time log, try to be as specific and as detailed as possible.

It shouldn't be surprising that time tracking apps are commonly available. *Hubstaff, HoursTracker, TrackingTime, Timely,* and *Hours* are just a few which offer different functions for tracking your time and the time of your staff, if you have one. Apps and websites which specialize in corporate time tracking for office management include

Paymo, Paydirt, Toggle, TimeTiger, Zoho, and others. Some of these apps are great for tracking budgetary and fiscal concerns as well.

Multitasking is one way we unconsciously procrastinate, for example. We think we're getting several things done, but none of them are being done as well as they could be, and studies prove that more mistakes are likely when focus is divided over several different tasks done at once. But that doesn't mean different tasks can't be done sequentially, one after the other. These are the tasks which get done successfully.

We've already seen how a strong support network can be an effective way to combat procrastination and overthinking. But a lot of people tend (unconsciously or not) to keep their professional and personal networks isolated. While there can be benefits to this, there are advantages to intermingling them as well. Friends can offer professional connections, and coworkers can become close friends.

OVERCOMING YOUR NEGATIVE SELF-TALK & PROCRASTINATION GOES HAND IN HAND

Negative self-talk, including self-blame and self-shame, self-deprecation, anything that breaks down your image of yourself. It's one of the great methods of self-sabotage and key to understanding procrastination and overthinking.

Negative self-talk leads to depression, lost opportunities, limited thinking, perfectionism, and relationship challenges.

By this time, you'll probably recognize what's become the procrastinator's motto: "I have to finish this long, important project. It should already be done by now and I need to plow through it."

But this is the kind of self-talk that can only fuel the procrastination cycle. But if you break this down, every part of the motto itself propagates the procrastination itself! The motto begins with *I have to*, but that's already shouldering the task with a lot of unpleasant associations. Nobody likes doing something they have to do. And there's an air of servitude to it, and nobody likes to feel like a servant. Instead, replace that with *I choose to*, which is far more empowering.

The motto goes on to use the word *finish*, but that only makes the task seem like one big thing. Instead, using the word *start* initiates a step-by-step process which can be more easily managed. In the same way, the long task should be reconsidered as a short task. If you're breaking the big job down into a series of smaller, more manageable tasks, then it *will* be a short task, right?

The motto's *important project* puts too much pressure on the performance and brings out the perfectionist protagonist in anyone. And since you've broken the big job down into smaller tasks, each one needn't be perfect for the whole to be a success. The *important project* becomes an *imperfect step*.

The motto goes on to say, *it should have been done by now*, and that may be true. But the verbiage is loaded with negativity. It implies failure and can only damage the worker's self-efficacy, a prime element of both procrastination and overthinking. Instead, replace that clause with *I'll feel terrific*. That's setting yourself a reward for accomplishment, an excellent motivator.

The motto closes with *I need to plow through it*. That establishes expectations of a long haul, which almost anybody would dread and then avoid. Instead, promise yourself, I'll have plenty of time for play. Again, you'll have something to look forward to, and you'll be looking ahead to long-term satisfaction instead of immediate gratification.

So, if the procrastinator's motto is, "I have to finish this long, important project. It should already be done by now and I need to plow through it," then let the non-procrastinator's motto be, "I choose to start this task with a small, imperfect step. I'll feel terrific and have plenty of time for play!"

Another kind of destructive self-talk is low self-compassion. The people that are hardest on themselves are less likely to be as productive as they could be. It's counterintuitive, because one might imagine that those who drive themselves harder would be more productive, but the resultant feelings of failure actually create the opposite effect. It creates stress and stress is harmful for the health and productivity of the worker, as we've seen.

Instead, practice self-compassion (few will offer you their compassion, after all). Forgive yourself for you mistakes or shortcomings, understand that you're doing your best and that nobody and nothing is perfect. But you have to do it deliberately. Self-compassion is the easiest thing to forget. You may have heard the old phrase, "We're hardest on ourselves." Well, make a conscious effort not to do that, and you'll be a lot happier, healthier, and more productive. Here's another old one: Guy goes to a doctor, bends his arms backward, and says, "Doc, it hurts when I do this." The doctor replies, "Then don't do that."

Of course, it's not always that easy. If you're plagued by negative self-talk, try asking yourself, "What am I feeling right now? Self-blame, self-shame? Am I indulging in negative self-talk?" If you are, don't do that. Instead, do the opposite and indulge in some positive self-talk. "Good job, buddy! Doin' great, sister!"

If that doesn't help, try something like, "May I be safe in this moment, may I be secure and accepted and loved." Don't forget to breathe in a deep, slow, steady rhythm. Then choose to do something which will bring you something pleasant and nurturing to put you back on track for more productivity later. But give yourself time to slow down and recalibrate.

To combat negative self-talk, learn to identify your inner critic and don't simply submit to it. Give it a nickname, like Debbie Downer or Mr. Grumpy Pants. Reduce its power over you and don't let the inner critic be constantly on your back. Stand up to them, cross-examine them, put their negativity to the test and you may just see it fall apart under scrutiny. He or she isn't real, after all. Thoughts aren't reality.

You can also set boundaries, even for yourself. Make it clear to your inner critic that some subjects are off-limits. You may also be conscious of negative language and replace it with neutral language. Replace "I hate …" with "I don't like …" Replace "I can't stand this …" with "This is a big challenge." Negative language fosters negative thoughts. Words have meaning.

You may consider replacing your inner critic with an inner friend, one who naturally frames things in a positive fashion. Your inner critic may say, "You're worthless!" But your inner friend will say, "You're precious worthy!" Your inner critic may claim that you've fallen behind and failed in life, but your inner friend will reassure you that you still have so many accomplishments ahead of you.

You may reconsider your perspective. Will what's upsetting you now mean anything to anyone in five years? Does it affect anyone outside of your immediate circle? If not, maybe it's not such a big deal to generate all that negative self-talk.

And don't be afraid to say these things out loud. We've already seen how talking to somebody or even to yourself can be cathartic and helpful, and it works here as well. Give voice to it and that gives your new perspective even more power. Your ears will hear it, and that will help your brain to believe it.

It can be as easy as simply saying the word *stop!* When the negative self-talk begins, just tell yourself to stop, insist on it. Imagine a stop sign, or a door slamming shut to end the negative internal conversation.

Here's another interesting equation: *Events + Thoughts = Emotions.* An event strikes a person as troubling and they emotionally react. So, in essence, thoughts mediate emotions. You can't change the events, but if you want to control your emotional reactions, you need only change your thoughts.

But these thoughts don't occur in a vacuum. And there are general mistakes negative self-talkers make which only feeds the cycle of procrastination and overthinking.

Mindreading is the tendency to make assumptions about what others are thinking. These assumptions are almost always wrong, but they can be the subject of unending negative self-talk. Imagine being on a date and the other seems reserved. You may upset yourself with the certainty of a rejection, or it could be simple shyness.

Overgeneralizing is the tendency to assume that isolated events will repeat in a pattern. If the one date didn't go well, one may assume no date ever will. Fortune telling makes a similar error in perspective.

Magnification makes every unpleasant event a catastrophe. That date will be remembered as the worst date in history, and that will only propagate negative self-talk and limit future opportunities based on overgeneralizing.

Minimization is the other side of that coin, reducing every pleasant experience to coincidence or luck, but not due to personal achievement. Minimizing reduces the person as well as the event. The date may have gone well, but that could be attributed to a free meal, right?

Emotional reasoning allows a person to make decisions based on feelings instead of facts. Maybe the date went well, but this person just doesn't feel the right attraction or allows nervousness or fear of failure to prevent further engaging.

Black and white thinking leads us to exaggerate the nature of people and events to one extreme or the other. A bad date leads some to believe that dating itself is bad.

Black and white thinking often leads to personalization, when those extremes are applied to the self-talker, who takes too much responsibility for events outside of their control. The unfortunate dater may feel that he failed to charm his companion, when it could just as easily be something beyond their control. Some people just won't date others for a variety of reasons; race, height, other things nobody can control.

Labelling naturally results from all this negative self-talk. After the bad date, one may call themselves a loser. That's not a label anybody should have to wear.

Using the word *should* can be destructive too. It leads to overthinking about the past and the future, but that only stifles events in the present, as we've seen.

You can look for these mistakes in others' behavior as well as your own. You won't be able to control what others think and say, but you'll be able to avoid them and use other skills we've discussed in this book to better deal with them. Ask positive questions to counter the negative statements, for example.

And if you must be self-critical, do it intentionally and not habitually. It will give your self-critiques more validity and more effectiveness.

We talked about self-compassion, which is really a kind of positive self-talk. And just as there are drawbacks to negative self-talk, there are benefits to positive self-talk, including an increased life span, lower rates of distress and depression, better psychological and physical wellbeing, better cardiovascular health, improved coping skills and resistance to stress, even greater resistance to the common cold (still no cure though).

Positive thoughts flood your brain with endorphins, encouraging relaxation and contributing to alertness and a more centered psyche.

To encourage positive self-talk, consider identifying areas to improve, be conscious of your daily thoughts, embrace humor and a healthy lifestyle, surround yourself with positive people, and deliberately practice self-compassion and positive self-talk. It's easier than you think!

THE TRUTH ABOUT DOPAMINE, AND HOW TO 'HACK' YOUR BRAIN TO MAKE DOING 'HARD TASKS' SO MUCH EASIER (YOU MIGHT EVEN FIND YOURSELF STARTING TO ENJOY THEM)

Dopamine is a neurotransmitter produced in your body and used by the nervous system to transmit messages between nerve cells. Dopamine influences how we think and plan, strive and focus and find things interesting or pleasurable.

Studies show a connection between dopamine and several behavioral or biological functions, such as motivation, learning, heart rate, kidney and blood vessel function, sleep and mood and attention, lactation, and processing pain or nausea.

Too little dopamine has been related to schizophrenia, ADHD, and drug use and addiction.

Dopamine may be created by the body as a result of pleasure or even in anticipation of it, triggered by related sights and smells.

Symptoms of dopamine deficiency include difficulty concentrating, reduced motivation, concentration, enthusiasm, and alertness, poor coordination and challenged movement. Conditions associated with low dopamine levels include depression, Parkinson's disease, and dopamine transporter deficiency syndrome, or infantile parkinson-ism-dystonia, which causes uncontrolled movements similar to Parkinson's.

But too much dopamine isn't a good thing either. It can cause hallucinations, delusions, and mania and is associated with addiction, obesity, and schizophrenia.

If you're low on dopamine, there are a variety of ways to boost your levels.

Consider a change of diet to foods rich in tyrosine. These include meats, cheese, fish, soy, dairy, nuts, seeds, lentils, and beans. You can try a tyrosine supplement as well. You can increase magnesium levels by eating more nuts, soy, seeds, beans, and whole grains.

Avoid high-fat foods, sugar, caffeine, and processed foods. Correct harmful sleep habits and exercise daily. Use meditation, breathing exercises, and visualization to avoid stress.

You may even try natural nootropics like L-theanine and L-Tyrosine.

Neuroplasticity is the process of change in the brain in response to repeated experiences. So, if you use the techniques you've learned in this book, such as indulging in positive thought and adopting a healthier lifestyle, you actually train your brain to create more dopamine.

Exercise and productivity are good ways to burn through excess dopamine.

The section of the brain associated with automatic emotional reaction is the amygdala. This is where the fight or flight response occurs in times of great pressure. Often, to fight is to resist, and to take flight may take the form of merely ignoring a certain person or event.

Norepinephrine is produced, creating increased fear and anxiety, then adrenalin only makes the feelings worse. Dopamine, on the other hand, is the pleasure communicator. Experts have found that, to beat procrastination and overthinking, it's helpful to have more dopamine and less norepinephrine.

Our technique of turning one big task into series of smaller tasks will help us achieve that. A smaller, completed task encourages the brain to produce dopamine, and that dopamine fuels our further efforts. Conversely, the stress of completing one huge task forestalls the reward and thus the dopamine while encouraging the production of norepinephrine. Once again, it's a matter of changing your behavior before you change your thinking.

GET RID OF YOUR IMPULSIVE BEHAVIOR AND STOP DELAYING THINGS, THE SECRET TO GETTING AHEAD IS GETTING STARTED, AND YOU ALREADY KNOW IT DEEP DOWN (SO STOP DENYING IT!)

Impulsive behavior is generally not well planned, rather it occurs in the spur of the moment without thought to the consequences. Different impulsive adult behaviors include binging on food, liquor, or drugs; destruction of property, as in a temper tantrum; escalating problems and arguments, frequent outbursts; self-harm like cutting; physical violence such as punching; oversharing too much about personal or inappropriate subjects, and higher-risk sex.

In children, look for ignoring danger, interrupting, vocal aggression, physical aggression and grabbing.

Impulsiveness may be caused by personality or learned experience, or brain connectivity or function, but one cannot rule out the influence of genetics, childhood trauma, genetics, or physical changes in the body.

Mental disorders such as ADHD, antisocial personality, intermittent explosive disorder, borderline personality and bipolar may contribute to impulsiveness as well. Kleptomania (the desire to steal), pyromania (the desire to burn), and trichotillomania (the desire to pull out your own hair) are closely associated with impulsive behavior. Pathological gambling is one of the classic impulsive behaviors.

Brain injury and stroke may be contributing factors as well.

But there are times when impulsive behavior can be remedied. With an adult, consider walking through the possible scenarios of what may happen as a consequence. Take a moment to really think it through. The same is good for impulsive behavior in a child, though making a role-play game of it may make the lesson sink in a bit more effectively. They're children, after all.

As before, the environment is crucial, as it has a tremendous influence. In this case, seek out the triggers of your impulsive behavior and change your environment to exclude them as much as you can. Impulsive gamblers should stay out of casinos, for example. Impulse eaters shouldn't walk past the bakery. Change where you go, change your route to work to avoid the bakery, and you'll thwart those triggers and be able to change your behaviors.

As we've seen, the best way to get something done is to get it started. The journey of a thousand miles begins with a single step, as they say. And we've seen the value of breaking a big task down to small, manageable tasks. Well, the first of those tasks can only be one thing; getting started. The old saying, which has been attributed to a variety of sources including Mark Twain, goes like this: The key to getting ahead is getting started.

So, follow Nike's advice and just do it. It doesn't have to be great; it just has to be. You can correct it later if you need to, but at least you'll be engaged in the task and not stymied by analysis paralysis.

A lot of this will require self-control, and that can be improved. Like any big project, break it down into manageable tasks. Pay your credit card on time and enjoy the feeling of being responsible. The ensuing dopamine will propel you into the next self-control task, counting the calories of your next meal. You'll feel better and stronger and encouraged to move on to your next task of self-control, a trip to the gym. It's an upward spiral instead of a downward spiral, and one with all the positive mental and physical benefits to help you live a better life. You'll find that impulse control, procrastination, and overthinking are basically issues of self-control as well. And once you've conscientiously increased your self-control, you'll find tackling those problems easier as well.

APPLY DELAYED GRATIFICATION, AND MAKE TASKS URGENT USING ACTIVE PROCRASTINATION

A big part of defeating the cycle of procrastination and overthinking is delaying gratification. Immediate gratification is one of the leading factors in procrastination, as we've seen. But there are significant benefits to delaying gratification.

A Stanford University placed children in a room with a plate holding a single marshmallow. They were told they could eat the treat or wait 15 minutes and get two marshmallows. The ones who waited generally also did better on standardized tests, better behavior, and better health.

In your case, the delayed gratification which comes at the completion of a big task will be all the sweeter, and well worth waiting for if you break it down simply. Delayed gratification is at least twice as good as immediate gratification, but really, it's a hundred times greater, incalculably greater.

Think about previous experiences when you didn't wait and went for immediate gratification. How did that make you feel, what did you take away from that experience. Now reflect on a time you did wait or had to wait, like Christmas Day. How do you remember those experiences? Wasn't Christmas Day all the sweeter, more precious, for the wait?

The study also showed that children who were told to picture the marshmallows as little fluffy clouds had an easier time waiting, and those who were asked to describe the flavor and sensation of eating the marshmallows were less willing to wait. This suggests that emotion is a greater impulse trigger than reason.

Delayed gratification can also deliver the motivational factor that immediate gratification simply can't. Delayed gratification creates a goal, something to work toward. But immediate gratification cannot do this by its very nature, because it's immediate and goals are at least slightly longer-term in nature.

Buying a house, retirement, getting married, these are classic goals and all of them entail delayed gratification.

It's very likely that delayed gratification improves with time and maturity. An adult is more likely to value delayed gratification than a child. Baumeister's 2007 self-control and self-regulation theory (Baumeister, 2007), describes five different areas or domains of gratification delay. They include food, physical pleasure, social interaction, money, and achievement.

It's hard to resist a tasty snack, for example (food), a nice backrub (physical pleasure), a fun night out (social interaction), a quick bet (money), or a quick laugh (achievement). But these are the areas where delay is the most beneficial. Delaying food is healthier, delaying physical pleasure can lead to greater pleasure later. Avoiding a quick bet will save you the loss, a quick laugh may be inappropriate. Delay is only natural in these domains, they're a natural part of these things. We wait until mealtime to eat, until it's an appropriate time and place for physical pleasure. We make dates to go out and prepare for that event. We receive paychecks in two-week increments. We get promotions after years of work. We *have* to wait for these things.

Procrastination does have some positive aspects; however, active procrastination can be turned to anyone's advantage if they understand what it is and how it works.

Procrastination helps a person to learn how to manage delays, provides chances to reflect on your course and often results in making better choices. Procrastination may aid in prioritization and allow for smaller chores to get done. In its strange way, procrastination is the antithesis of impulsive behavior.

It took naturalist Charles Darwin 20 years to finish *On the Origin of Species*. Renaissance genius Leonardo da Vinci spent years fussing with his Mona Lisa. He was a perfectionist procrastinator.

Studies of college students indicate that many procrastinators are more competitive and ego-driven, whereas non-procrastinators are more task-driven.

Most people think of procrastination as being essentially passive; after all, procrastination is all about *not* doing a certain task, right?

But there is an active form of procrastination, when someone postpones a task deliberately and diverts attention to more important tasks. Those who actively procrastinate seem to prefer working under pressure. They are motivated by the challenge and often succeed in meeting deadlines.

Active procrastination has three major facets. The first is cognitive, when a person decides to procrastinate. The second is affective, when a person prefers time pressure. The third is behavioral, wherein they still complete the task on time.

Active procrastination is closely associated with multi-tasking. Active procrastinators tend to use task-oriented coping strategies in times of stress, avoiding emotional reactions. Passive procrastinators lean toward avoidance-coping strategies and rely on emotional reactions. Active procrastinators are driven by both intrinsic motivation, which comes from within, and the extrinsic motivation of a looming deadline. Active procrastinators often have a significant level of autonomy, self-reliance, and self-confidence.

But active procrastination must be learned, and here's a good exercise to help you adapt the more beneficial type of procrastination. Set yourself a simple task, let's say sending an email. Then put yourself in the place where that task is done, which in this case would be in front of a computer. Now don't do it, wait as long as you dare. Feel the emotions which result from waiting, accept that it will be uncomfortable, boring, frustrating, stressful. Let the feelings come ... and then let them go. You need to deal from a rational place, not an emotional place. Once the feelings have passed, begin the task. You've now mastered your emotions, and that's something the passive protagonist struggles with. Now you're ready to complete the task and get that email written!

As we discussed earlier, a habit is easy to give up and hard to quit. So often the best recourse is to take up the opposite habit. Instead of giving up meat, become a vegetarian. And the same is true for passive procrastination. It's habitual and a hard habit to break. But you can choose to be an active procrastinator instead, and let the good habit simply replace the bad.

POMODORO, THE PROCRASTINATORS' NEW BEST FRIEND

We've already discussed the notion of breaking down one big task into several smaller tasks, and the various benefits to this approach. But a more precise version of this approach is called the *Pomodoro Technique.*

The Pomodoro Technique recommends breaking big tasks down into 25-minute chunks, with a break of about 5- or 10-minutes. The technique refers to these 25-minute work periods as *Pomodoros.*

The frequent breaks keep you refreshed and focused, and the careful measurement of time keeps you focused and disciplined, while completing each Pomodoro gratifies and brings the reward of self-satisfaction and positive self-efficacy.

The Pomodoro is best implemented in stages; planning, tracking, recording, processing, visualization. Plan the day's events at the beginning of the day. Track your progress and new information throughout the day. Make a record at the end of the day to see the results of your progress. Also, at the end of the day, process that data into information by visualizing it so you can understand it clearly and use it to your benefit later.

To implement the Pomodoro Technique, use a timer to make sure you stick to the schedule. Start with a to-do list, in order of priority, and include a section for unexpected interruptions. Keep an activity inventor sheet too, to mark these things down, and a records sheet to list the data compiled throughout the day. And don't skip the breaks, they're important to keep you focused and vital throughout the day. Breaks are well known to have a lot of benefits. They let you take a step back and re-evaluate, rev up your brain, think of better ideas, and prevent exhaustion.

PROVEN STRATEGIES THAT WILL HELP YOU BEAT YOUR PROCRASTINATION

One advanced technique to control procrastination is Eisenhower's Urgent/Important Principle, which emphasizes using time effectively and not simply efficiently. This technique helps you to prioritize, to differentiate which tasks on your to-do list are important and which are more like distractions.

Being effective and not merely efficient means breaking down activities into two groups. Important activities relate to long-term goals, whereas urgent activities have to be dealt with immediately but may not relate to anything long-term. Knowing the difference will help you prioritize between the two.

Try it for yourself! Make a list of everything you do during the day, no matter how inconsequential it may be. Then break those activities into four categories; important *and* urgent, important *but not* urgent, *not* important *but* urgent, and not important *and also not* urgent.

When things are important and urgent, they may include things which are scheduled (important) and things which are unplanned (urgent). You'll want to schedule extra time to accommodate both. Important but not urgent tasks are vital for long-term success, so make plenty of time for these in your daily schedule. When something is not important but urgent, think about delegating the task if your time is taken up by something, anything, which is important. When something is not important and also not urgent, put that at the bottom of the list and reschedule until there is nothing in the first three categories.

Another helpful tip for beating procrastination is to break down your sense of time to the smallest increment. Instead of looking at your deadline as being three days away, think of it as being in 72 hours. It gives the delay a sense of being shorter and adds urgency to your motivation.

Think about how your work affects others. Very often, we lack self-care and self-support, but we're very caring and giving to others. Remember the phrase, "We're always hardest on ourselves"? Well, this gets to the root of that. So instead of thinking about yourself and your efficacy or insecurity, think about the others around you. If you procrastinate, how will that affect them, their careers and reputations?

You might also recast the deadline. If it's due on a Monday, give yourself a deadline of the previous Friday so you're sure to get it done even if you do procrastinate a bit.

Publicly committing to the deadline is a good way to put the pressure on. It's like giving your word. Your integrity and standing are great motivators! A motivational friend to check in and support you is also a potent strategy. You might think about making a gentlemen's bet with somebody that you'll finish the task!

Another good exercise is to pick a small task and give yourself five minutes to finish it. That'll be one small victory for you, one small defeat for procrastination. A lot of people have a favorite song which gets them excited for a particular task. Music creates emotional responses, and emotions have great power to inspire our behavior, as we have seen.

Now that we've made considerable progress defeating procrastination, let's do the same thing with overthinking!

OVERCOME YOUR OVERTHINKING!

DECLUTTERING YOUR MIND HELPS YOU RECHARGE YOUR BRAIN & RE-SHAPE YOUR BEHAVIORS & HABITS IN AS LITTLE AS DAYS

Previously, we looked at how the environment can influence thought and behavior. And in just the same way one's environment can become cluttered, so too can the mind. But decluttering the mind is a great way to overcome your overthinking.

So, consider your mental furniture; does it fit, do pieces clash? Are your mental appliances all in good working order, so you can cook when you need to and cool down when you need to? Does the décor really reflect who you are now or is there a lot of old stuff it's time to replace.

And while we're looking at the correlation to mind and environment, take a look at your actual environment. Is your house clean? Is your desk cluttered? Are you well-organized? These things will affect your psyche as much as they are affected by them.

Writing down your concerns is a great way to get them out of your mind, because those thoughts are now being stored elsewhere. Journal keeping has this benefit and lots of others, including giving you a chance to organize the things you're overthinking about and then solving or resolving them, turning negative thought into positive behavior.

Mental clutter is often caused by memories of things past; not pleasant memories, but grudges and unpleasant events which could perhaps have worked out differently. Let go of those things in the same way you'd throw out old magazines. They're not contemporary or relevant to your life in the present, and they take up a lot of space.

Multi-tasking tends to lead to a lot of mental clutter, because too many things are being tended to at once and they all can't be done to complete satisfaction. Multi-tasking clutters the worker's time and as a result, it clutters their mind.

Too much information is perhaps the leading culprit of mental clutter, and that makes sense. In our world today, we get more information and faster than ever before. The news cycles are shorter, the array of information is ever widening. So naturally we have too much information. But how do we resist that in this hyper-informative age? Limit your time on the internet or in front of the TV, be discerning about what you pay attention to.

Being decisive is a good way to combat overthinking too, because decisive action replaces the overthought which may create analysis paralysis. Being decisive also helps you prioritize, another key to breaking the overthinking and procrastinating cycles.

One great way to clear mental clutter is to meditate, that's a big part of what meditation is all about; clearing your mind and focusing. Deep breathing is a big part of meditation, and that practice on its own can be very helpful in ridding your mind of clutter.

As you might do with procrastinating, think about finding a supportive friend to talk to about your concerns. Speaking them will help get them off your chest and off your mind.

A healthy sleep cycle is important to sound mental health, and that's a key to breaking the overthinking cycle. Wake up early and go to bed at a reasonable time. Avoid things which will disrupt your sleeping patterns, as we've already discussed.

Getting in touch with nature is a great way to alleviate mental clutter. It's another case of the connection between environment and mental health. Once again, change your environment and you can change your whole way of thinking. The sounds of birds singing, a babbling brook, wind blowing through the trees, the smells and sights of the woods or even a public park, are refreshing and calming and should go far to helping rid you of that mental clutter.

A lot of people keep a mental inventory, which is a list of things one must do, things one should do, things one wishes to do. Once they're stored elsewhere, you can take them off your mental desktop, so to speak. Ask yourself how important each item truly is, to you or someone close to you. Keep revising that inventory as necessary, as old tasks are completed and new ones come up.

The brain is responsible for a variety of neurological and cognitive function, the latter group including language, attention, memory, visual-spatial skills, and executive function. But the brain can become bored with these functions and needs frequent stimulation. You can use specific challenges and relaxation acts to keep the brain functioning at its best.

Learning a new skill can be both a challenge and a relaxation act. Learning to cook, to paint, or play a musical instrument are great to both challenge and relax. Therapeutic yoga is also both challenging and relaxing, and very good for the body. Getting plenty of rest is a relaxation act (and often a challenge too) but it's vital to refresh the brain.

Problem-solving activities like puzzles and video games are a good way to keep the brain stimulated and eager to process new data. Expressing yourself artistically, as we mentioned earlier, is a great way to relax; dance, journaling, singing. It doesn't matter how good you're at these things either. This is not the time to be a perfectionist!

And don't forget to take time off for things you enjoy, as this balance is vital for an uncluttered and refreshed mind.

5 EASY STRATEGIES FOR OVERCOMING PERFECTIONISM & HOW THIS WILL REDUCE YOUR OVERTHINKING

Perfectionism, the drive to perform and produce flawlessly, may seem like a strong motivator, but we've already seen how it can actually impede productivity. It can also contribute to a lot of negative conditions, including depression, anxiety, obsessive-compulsive disorder, burnout, eating disorders, and suicide risk.

We've already seen that it's one of the major contributors to procrastinating and to overthinking as well. No conversation would ever have been perfect, no possible situation will ever be perfect. Nothing will ever be perfect, and if they are, that's probably owed to a dash of luck, something nobody can control.

As we did before, let's take a look at the language we use, because words have meaning and can drastically change our perspectives. For example, a perfectionist might say, "I didn't get an A on a test; I'm a complete failure." But an alternative might be something like, "Whatever the grade is, will it matter a year from now?" The perfectionist may say, "My haircut looks awful, I don't want to be seen." But the alternative may be something like, "People have bigger things to worry about, and it'll always grow back. With the way people wear their hair these days, probably nobody will even notice."

The attitudes are completely different, and so too will be the resultant behaviors.

But here are 5 concrete ways to help overcome your perfectionist overthinking:

- First, make a list of the advantages and disadvantages of trying to be perfect. You'll see right away how dangerous the disadvantages are (relationship problems, anxiety) and the advantages (better decisions after clearer reflection).
- Second, be more self-aware. If you tend toward perfectionism, substitute those thoughts with more humble thoughts. Focus on the positive in a project, not the inevitable little flaws.
- Third, as with procrastination, set a time schedule with limits and stick to it. It's a matter of self-control and self-care.
- Fourth, learn not to see criticism as a personal attack, don't respond to it defensively. Listen to the criticism and don't counter it, just digest it. If you've made a mistake, acknowledge it but don't beat yourself up for it. Everybody has the right to make a mistake now and then. Nobody's perfect, right?
- Fifth, set reasonable goals which you can accomplish. Setting huge goals which may be next to impossible is virtually setting yourself up for failure and disappointment, fueling the overthinking cycle.

A word about goal setting here. Perfectionists tend to set certain goals which only feed the perfectionist tendencies. Non-perfectionists set goals of a different sort. For instance, perfectionists often set goals based on what others expect. A healthier goal is based on personal wants or desires. Perfectionists believe their goal is perfection, while a healthier goal is based on relativity to the worker's abilities or recent achievements. The perfectionist may set a goal with the focus on the end result, while a healthier goal setting system may emphasize the pleasure to be found in the process; creativity and working with others, forming bonds, and so on. The perfectionist fears disapproval or failure as connected to the self, but a healthier goal setting mindset associates disapproval or failure with the project, not the workers.

And, when you're setting your goals, don't forget to be SMART. The goals should be specific, measurable, achievable, realistic, and timely; SMART.

Another good way to prevent perfectionism is to try to see a problem through somebody else's eyes. What would they make of it? What advice would you give to them? Remember, we're hardest on ourselves.

An exposure technique is when a person faces, or exposes themselves, to their greatest fear in order to conquer that fear. For the protagonists, those fears include rejection, failure, ridicule. So, a perfectionist can always deliberately achieve a little failure in order to discover how non-catastrophic such a thing could be. It may sound strange (unthinkable to some) but go ahead and mess up a little bit. Drop your train of thought during a presentation or wear a wrinkled shirt. Let an awkward pause go for a while longer than you might have. Then sit back and see what happens ... which will probably be nothing. Imperfections really only bother the perfectionist, and that's a vital lesson to learn to curb that often-destructive trait.

Another neat trick in dealing with perfectionism is to get a new hobby. You're not likely to master it right away, so you won't be expecting perfection ... hopefully. You'll be more drawn into the moment of learning and growing and not in the results or their consequences.

CULTIVATE YOUR MENTALITY TO ITS PEAK PERFORMANCE AND RELIEVE YOURSELF FROM ANXIETY AND NEGATIVE THOUGHTS

Perfectionists aren't the only ones who have anxiety and fear of failure, of course. We've already looked at some coping mechanisms for fear of failure and other problems common to procrastination and overthinking; be aware of the causes and triggers, reframe your beliefs around the goal to deemphasize the consequences, change your language and perspective from the negative to the positive, visualize potential outcomes, consider the worst-case scenario, and have a backup plan. Whatever happens, learn from it for the next time!

Ask yourself what you learned from a certain situation, how you can grow as a result of it, and find at least three positive things from the experience.

A SOUND MIND IS IN A SOUND BODY

We've talked about healthy and unhealthy diets and their effects on sound mental health, procrastination, and overthinking. The central organ of overthinking, the brain, has an even stronger connection to the body. The brain never stops working, not for one second during your life. So, it requires an incredible amount of energy, more than any other part of the body.

In fact, brain cells consume twice the energy of other cells. At between only two and three percent of the average person's body mass, the brain burns a full 20% of calories consumed.

So healthy diet and lifestyle are crucial for the brain, and for the cognitive functions the brain controls, as we've discussed. They provide the long-lasting mental agility needed to be productive. Ever have a big meal and then sort of crash? It's because overeating floods the brain with too much glucose. Too little glucose has a similar, debilitating effect.

Processed foods which are sugary, salty, or fatty take longer for the body to digest (a full three days for a McDonald's Big Mac). And that means less useful fuel for the brain ... and the rest of the body too.

For optimal mental and physical health, experts recommend avoiding anything processed, and eating your organic or natural foods slower to aid digestion. Your stomach takes about 15 minutes to send the message to your brain that you're full. Eating faster means you fill that gap with more food than you need, flooding your brain with glucose.

A few tips and tricks to eating healthier include substituting meats for vegetables in dishes like pizza or an omelet. Take coffee or tea without cream and sugar. Veggies and hummus can replace chips and dip at your next party. Cook at home, it tastes better and you know exactly what's in it and the circumstances under which it was made. If takeout is a lifestyle necessity, find the healthiest options. Taco Bell? Try

Subway. KFC? Well, anything's probably better than KFC unless you just eat the box. Even then ...

Running is an exercise and a recreational pastime which can have terrific advantages to a sound body and mind. It burns calories, builds circulatory and cardiovascular health, but studies show it offers brain support and enhances mood. It calms the mind as we concentrate on the basic movement instead of more complicated intellectual concerns. Running also uses up excess adrenaline or cortisol to diffuse stress.

Any exercise should be done in moderation, of course. Experts recommend 20-30 minutes at a time, two to three times a week.

Use a lot of the same techniques you used for procrastination (healthy sleep and diet, self-compassion, reflection, depersonalization) to help overcome your overthinking. And don't just think about it, do it!

SETTING GOALS THAT ACTUALLY INSPIRE YOU & ARE BUILT ON YOUR DEEPEST DESIRES

The great artist Pablo Picasso once said, "Our goals can only be reached through a vehicle of a plan, in which we must fervently believe, and upon which we must vigorously act. There is no other route to success."

So, have a goal which has a plan you believe in and act on. That really doesn't sound so hard, but there are facets of it which are easy to overlook. One of those is the goal. We've already discussed the use of short-term goals to achieve a single long-term goal by breaking up a project into a series of smaller tasks. But it's important to set the right goals, to be smart, or SMART (right?) about selecting our goals.

WHY SMART GOALS ARE NOT ENOUGH TO NUDGE YOU

You'll recall that SMART is an acronym for goals which are specific, measurable, achievable, results oriented, and time bound. But setting good goals alone won't do it. You'll need to put them into action. You'll have broken the project down into smaller units which can be achieved, sometimes called *milestones*.

To put this into play, start by making a list of tasks which will achieve each milestone. Use a timeline for this, as we've discussed.

We've already talked about apps for time management, but they have them for goal setting too! GTD Agenda (Getting Things Done) is one, and the basic $4.45-per-month plan allows you to track up to 30 goals and 50 tasks! *GoalsOnTrack*, *Profit*, *ClearCompany*, *7Geese*, *Lattice*, *Sprigg*, and *Wrike* are others.

Because while smart (or SMART) goals are great, goal setting can be a lot more involved. Goals are not only crucial to the basic pattern of accomplishment, the first crucial step in that cycle, but studies have shown that they increase motivation and organization. And the more challenging and the more valuable the goal, the greater our efforts will be to achieve it and the greater the results of success will be.

Studies also show that clearly defined goals will lead to a superior performance. Research has produced a theory of goal setting based off five key principles: Commitment, clarity, challenge, complexity, feedback.

It really only makes perfect sense. The more committed we are to a task, the more likely we are to access and achieve. Commitment comes from proper motivation, such as long-term gain. Conversely, lack of commitment inspires lesser results, especially when the task is a challenging one.

Clarity is also key; the nature and purpose of the task, its value, its deadline. If a worker is confused as to what they're doing or why they're doing it, that greatly increases the chances of failure and inhibits the likelihood of achievement. But who could commit to something they can't even understand?

It's easy to see how these steps, like many in such equations, lead from one right into the other.

Once you have commitment and clarity, the goal should be challenging. It shouldn't be impossible, clearly, but boring and mundane tasks are the least appealing to the human psyche and most encouraging of negative mindsets which cause procrastination and overthinking. The human being likes to be challenged; it's how we built the pyramids and put a man on the Moon.

Complexity is important, as it must come in moderation. Challenge is great, but too much complexity interrupts the clarity we need to get the tasks done. But complexity does occur, often unforeseen and as a result of the accomplishing of the task itself, so make sure to budget a bit more time into a project timeline to account for complexity.

Feedback keeps the process and the progress moving forward during each of these stages.

A bit more on goals and how to set them:

Goal setting has been shown to improve academic performance up to 25%. Setting the right goal has been associated with optimal *flow state*, or *being in the zone*, as they say.

Research on college students found that optimism and hope made students better suited to setting goals and achieving their tasks. Students with high self-efficacy did better than those with less self-confidence. Either type of student seems more likely to be influenced by social forces in setting their goals.

So far, we've talked about goal setting as a more-or-less individual practice, but with bigger projects which require teams, a team approach to goal setting can be an invaluable approach! Research has proven this, but it only stands to reason. People inspire one another and come up with better ideas, and that encourages higher morale, clearer positive thinking, better results, in an upward spiral. This is often a worksite experience, face-to-face, but the same principle applies to virtual teams, who must do their collaborating over Zoom. But musical combos are playing together over such devices, theatrical productions are being staged all over the internet, even *Saturday Night Live* has done it. So can you!

Virtual groups should consider having a sort of director to centralize communications and keep things on track.

Before any goals are set, remember that the practice requires planning (knowing what the task requires for completion and how to break it down conceptually), self-motivation (we have to want to achieve the goals we're setting), time management skills (budgeting how long each smaller goal will take to achieve), flexibility (to adjust for complexity), self-regulation (to ensure effective performance throughout the entire task), commitment and focus (to know what you want and how to get it).

There are also different areas related to goal setting. Know which area you're treading, and you'll be better equipped to set the right goals.

Researchers identify two types of achievement goals; mastery achievement goals (focusing on skill development to achieve the goal) and performance achievement goals (focusing on ability of the individual). Basically, mastery is about the result, performance is about the performer.

Mastery goals tend to inspire workers to complete the task. Their focus is on the qualities of the task, not of the worker. They work hard to improve their skills, to master them, in the cause of the task, especially in times of failure. Performance goals tend to orient individuals to prove themselves. Results are often personalized and reflect on the qualities of the worker, not the results of the task.

Performance goals can inspire anxiety and reduce task performance, but mastery goals can increase involvement through ongoing improvement and self-evaluation. So, mastery goals can have a more positive influence on motivation and that influences goal achievement.

But not all research agrees. Results of one study show that mastery goals worked well for those with low achievement orientation, but performance goals reduced those subjects' interest in the task, leading to poor performances. On the other hand, high achievement-oriented subjects had positive reactions to their performance-focused goals.

Some research suggests that performance goals should be subdivided into two approaches; *independent* and *avoidance orientations.* When setting goals, individuals are driven either by a desire for success or a fear of failure.

As long as we're breaking up one big task (goal setting) into smaller ones, let's look at three helpful categories of goals. Time goals categorize into two smaller groups; short-term and long-term goals. Focus goals are the big ones, they're the ultimate long-term goals. Topic-based goals are generally things which happen alongside but as a part of the task. Paying your bills or filing your taxes may be one of these but would a long-term goal like buying a home.

A good exercise, as we've discussed but it's worth repeating, is to set a few short-term goals and then achieve them. That begins a healthy cycle of success to motivate you to move on to bigger tasks and likewise accomplish them.

Then build on that task. Do one task in a day, then set three for the week, ten for the month, and so on. Be realistic, but challenge yourself! It'll be worth it even if you don't do all ten in the month. You'll have done five or seven, and that's a lot. The old saying goes, *"I'd rather strive for a lot and achieve half, than strive for nothing and achieve it all."*

YOUR INSPIRATIONS AND DEEPEST DESIRES WILL GIVE THE REAL PUSH THAT YOU NEED

Desire is a powerful emotion and an even more powerful motivator. It's also a tremendous force for creativity. So, it only makes sense to plumb those desires to achieve our goals.

Desire and the energy it generates have a huge influence on our intentions and on our actions. But desire may be so close to fear that they become indistinguishable. Often when we think we're moving toward we want (desire), we are often moving away from something we don't want (fear).

Fear motivation focuses avoiding penalties for failure and can lead to feelings of compulsion or inhibition. Desire motivation is focused on rewards for success but can lead to low self-efficacy and feelings of helplessness.

So, know the difference between what is motivating your goal setting, and lean toward the desire and away from the fear.

GOAL SETTING STRATEGIES THAT WORK LIKE MAGIC

Making a plan is always a good way to encourage results. As we've seen, say it or write it down and it will tend to take on its own life, become its own motivating factor. Some researchers think of this as an *implementation intention,* and that makes some sense. It's your stated intention to imply your plan to achieve your goal.

But this is best broken down to specific, smaller tasks. Try this exercise and write this down on a piece of paper, filling in the blanks according to your specific desires or goals:

> I will [BEHAVIOR] at [TIME] in [LOCATION].
>> Some examples are:
> I will sit in silence for five minutes at 6:30 a.m. in my
>> bed before getting up.
> I will study French for ten minutes at 8 p.m. in my
>> bedroom.
> I will go to the gym for one hour at 5 p.m. on
>> Mondays, Wednesdays, and Fridays.

Once you fall into the habit of doing these things regularly, they won't seem like chores, but a natural part of your routine. Eventually, they'll be the kind of habits you won't be able to quit, and you won't want to.

But let's be honest, it all may not work out perfectly; as we've seen, it's rare that anything does. So, if you hit a stumbling block and can't make habitual one of your chosen planned activities, think about using the *if/then* approach.

Make a new list, stating the same goal which may not have worked out before. Then add an if/then function to the sentence:

> If I sit in silence for five minutes at 6:30 a.m. in my bed
>> before getting up, then I'll have a better day.
> If I study French for ten minutes at 8 p.m. in my

bedroom, I'll have a better time on my trip when I finally go.

If I go to the gym for one hour at 5 p.m. on Mondays, Wednesdays, and Fridays, then I'll look great on my trip to France.

Here's another run through of the if/then principle, also quite practical:

If I don't sit in silence for five minutes at 6:30 a.m. in my bed before getting up, then I'll do it at the beginning of my lunch break, precisely at 12:00 noon.

If I don't study French for ten minutes at 8 p.m. in my bedroom, I'll do it in the car on my ride to work.

If I don't go to the gym for one hour at 5 p.m. on Mondays, Wednesdays, and Fridays, then I'll go for two hours on Saturday and Sunday.

This approach allows for the complexity of things to intrude on your carefully planned goals. Give yourself a backup plan and you'll be much more likely to get the goal set and the task done.

The *if/then* approach can be directly applied to the overarching problem of procrastination. To wit:

If I'm at my computer, then I'm working on the task. Otherwise, I'm somewhere else.

If I want to procrastinate, then I'll remind myself how

good it will feel to get the task done and all the
good the accomplishment of the long-term goal
would do for me.

One overlooked aspect to goal setting which we should touch on here is known as *calling a halt*. While we've been focused on setting our goals and achieving them, it's important to recall one of the benefits of overthinking, and that's a chance to re-evaluate. Sometimes a goal which seems well-chosen proves out not to be the best choice. Sometimes a project is simply heading in the wrong direction. In that case, the team may need to recalibrate. Goals may need to be reconsidered. So, don't be afraid to call a halt to things, pull back and reconsider.

In setting a goal, you may consider creating a mantra. Anything simple enough to repeat over and over and which will support your mindset will work: *"I can do this, I can do this ..."* or "Everything's okay, everything's okay ..." I personally combat a fear of driving over bridges by singing a mangled version of a classic Pink Floyd song: "All in all you're just another stretch of the road." Vocalizing gives power, after all, and helps focus.

Here's another helpful acronym for setting goals and getting tasks done! WAVE stands for Write, Act, Visualize, Evaluate. We've already touched on all three, but acronyms are great ways to remember things. Pretty SMART, right?

Don't forget that goal setting is something we all do in every part of our lives; social, professional, creative, emotive. Setting goals can help improve all of these, when used effectively and not just efficiently.

SKYROCKET YOUR PRODUCTIVITY LEVEL

FOCUS ON WHAT YOU'RE GOOD AT, AND BECOME BETTER ON IT

We've all heard of multi-tasking, the practice of doing several things at once. We've looked into it here and found it to be less than effective in most cases. Odd, though, that the original concept of single tasking now seems more like the novelty than the norm. Our lives have become so dense with information and tasks and a dearth of time almost force us to multi-task, creating failed tasks, less self-efficacy, depression, and so on.

Single tasking allows you to focus, to get into the zone for optimal performance. Multi-tasking clearly prevents that, as it's a result of sharp focus and nobody can focus as sharply on three things simultaneously as well as they can on one thing at a time.

So now we have to train ourselves to return to our simpler recent past and retrain ourselves to be single taskers. This may be a challenge, but it is well within your ability.

First, as we've said, start with small tasks you can reasonably accomplish. Then make sure you only do one of them, and don't even consider another until you've finished the first. Then proceed to the next task following the same rule. The key here is not to set aside a task, not to begin another or to tend to any external event.

Don't forget to break the task down into reasonable, smaller goals.

With your daily to-do list, do them separately and do the most important task first. This way, you'll have little to dread for the rest of the day. Do the next more difficult chore second, and the rest of the day will get easier and easier.

As with other techniques toward related conditions and corrections, work in blocks of time and schedule breaks. And keep an uncluttered desk for an uncluttered mind. This is particular important when retraining to be a single tasker, as distractions and complexities will rise up and challenge your focus on that single task.

Despite all the focus we've put on setting realistic goals and deadlines, when it comes to retraining to be a single tasker, it may be better to set *un*realistic deadlines. *Harvard Business Review's* Peter Bergman suggests that limiting time available for a single task at a third of what might be expected normally. The notion is that the time will exert pressure enough to force completion by keeping the worker more focused. This may make workers more productive and far less stressed-out.

If you're working on a project which requires a lot of research, use some kind of placeholder in all caps (*RESEARCH*, for example), and then do all the research in one clump at the end of the day. Alternating between writing and research may seem like two parts of the same task, but a lot of time is lost going in and out of the zone, recalibrating from one skill set to the other and back. And it's really just multi-tasking of another sort, if you really think about it.

Also, while doing legitimate internet research for your project, you may be tempted to succumb to the distractions of email, videos, and other things which inhibit productivity.

Be mindful of the fulfillment you enjoy by fulfilling a task. When that's a single task, the feeling comes sooner and can inspire you to more productivity. And when you're doing this single task, don't succumb to perfectionism. Let the task go when it's done and move on to the next... after a bit of a break, of course.

And once you've set about to become a single tasker, considering limiting that one task to do the thing you do best.

It makes sense on a lot of levels. We all want to spend our time doing what we enjoy, and those are almost always the things we're good at. All the great businessmen, innovators, artists, and athletes in history were doing what they did best, after all. And wouldn't the project, the company, all of society be better off if we all did what we loved?

It might be, but life's just not like that. We have to do things we don't like, things we're not particularly great at doing; that's a big reason why we procrastinate. So, a sound business model to fighting procrastinating and find the thing you're best at, master it, and apply that mastery. This is a personal journey each and every one of us must take on our own, and woe to those who don't take it at all.

You may want to volunteer at work or outside of work to give yourself time and space to indulge in your special skills. This will help develop them and also bring them to the attention of others, those who may allow you to use those skills at the center of your productive life. Volunteering is good for self-efficacy, high self-esteem, physical and mental health, a widening social circle, and it has a variety of other benefits too.

Don't be afraid to take a compliment. There's no shame in being good at something, and you may even learn about a hidden skill you didn't know you had. People generally don't see us the same way we see ourselves, and procrastinators and overthinkers are notoriously hard on themselves.

Scarcity Mindset is described as the fear of expunging one's resources and losing all. It manifests itself in a lack self-efficacy, when you may harbor self-limiting beliefs and negative self-talk. So, there's an impulse to hoard due to a lack of confidence in the ability to earn. It's a self-perpetuating phenomenon because it creates over-workers who earn less, and this only reinforces the scarcity mindset.

But you can always move past it just by recognizing it and changing your perspective. Stop imagining that the worst is certain to come, that failure is certain. Neither is true.

It's interesting (and a bit sad) to note that a lot people just haven't found what their given gift or gifts are, what they're truly best at. A lot of people go from endeavor to endeavor, school to school, career to career, never really finding their niche. If that's you, you'll want to take concrete steps to finding that special thing at which you excel.

Ask yourself, *"What skills have helped me thrive?"* Are you the type who always has a funny quip, is that your defense mechanism to avoid a variety of uncomfortable situations? Well, there's an old saying among comics: *"Funny is money."* You might be better suited to a position where writing is central. Are you a person who pushes forward no matter what, imbued with a determination that nobody stands in your way? You might be better suited to a career as a first responder than a librarian.

Ask yourself, *"What makes me feel strong?"* If it's bringing a smile to a child's face, a career in teaching may suit you better than a career in construction. If helping old people gives you that special feeling, then you'll know where to volunteer. If playing violin has always been your secret passion, go play it at the local retirement home.

You may ask yourself, *"What made me stand out as a child?"* So often, we lose touch with the things which were most special about our childhood. Were you an imaginative kid? Maybe that's where your true skills are.

Of course, there is often a big difference between what you're good at and what you're passionate about. It's great if those two things intertwine, but it's not always the case. My father was passionate about opera but could never write or sing in one. Lots of people are passionate sports fans but could never even think of playing professionally. Conversely, a person may have a certain skill at math, but not be passionate about their job as a mid-level accountant. Or you may have passion for something you're good at and then lose passion for it. This kind of burnout it common to teachers, social workers, and those in the mental health field. So be careful to know what you're good at, what you're passionate about, and which ones will truly help you to progress.

You may assume the answer is to choose what you're good at rather than what you're passionate about, but that's not always so (few things are). True, they say to lean to your strengths, and that makes sense. Do what you know. It makes good sense though it can also be a limiting mindset, keeping a person in the same, basically unsatisfying position for years. Doesn't sound like a very happy life, does it?

On the other hand, you can learn new skills in line with your passions, after all. Passionate about food but can't open a restaurant? Learn a little bit about writing or video directing and think about being a food critic. You may not know much about how to captain a powerboat, but if you long to live in a small yacht, you can learn those things.

Your secret skill could also be associated with your environment. Did you grow up with some special cultural influences which might impact your work for the better? Did you grow up hunting alligators in the swamps? You might write a book about applying the skills of the alligator hunter to those of the modern young corporate up-and-comer. Or you might lend your passion for nature to environmental causes, that's a win/win for everybody (and everything).

To this end, remember that it's better to be great at one thing than fair at several. Once you find the skill which will propel you forward, devote yourself to it and exclude distractions. Greatness comes from mastery, and mastery comes from a lifetime of diligence and hard work. Mastery is your long-term goal once you've found your special skill, not immediate gratification. Avoid the pitfalls of procrastination and overthinking when your special skill is involved; you can't afford to let that opportunity pass you by.

WHY SAYING NO TO PEOPLE AND CERTAIN PROJECTS CAN HELP YOU GET A LOT MORE DONE

Saying *no* isn't as easy as it seems. In fact, it can be quite difficult. In this people-pleasing world, nobody wants to offend anybody else. And since most people don't like hearing the word, they assume others don't as well, and they're generally right. *Yes,* is just so much easier.

But sometimes you need to say *no*. This whole book is about saying *no*, in fact; *no* to negative thinking and self-talk, *no* to being locked helplessly in analysis paralysis, *no* to unhealthy living. But those things weren't easy. And it only gets harder from there.

Saying *no* to others means risking rejection, isolation, ultimate failure. For the perfectionist protagonist, the word *no* hits them at the very core of their being, it's not merely a rejection of the project or task but an absolute rejection of everything they are, were, or ever hope to be. That's a shame, but not only does it not have to be that, but *no* can be a very positive thing. It sounds counter-intuitive, but it's true. Let's take a closer look at when and how to say *no!*

If you have to say to others, a basic rejection of an offer or suggestion, there are ways to make it more comfortable for everyone involved.

You might cushion it with kindness or a compliment. Always start with something good, such as, *"You've done a lot of work on this, and I admire that. Thank you."* Or you might try to find the one good thing you can start with. *"I like the way you've organized these tasks."* Then move on to your suggestion, correction, or rejection.

Then give your reasons for saying no, if you must. Explain it in a way which takes the focus off the other person. Instead of saying, *"You're just not right,"* consider saying, *"We're going to go a different way with it."*

Be brief during these exchanges, but there's no reason to rush or be brusque. There's time enough to make sure you've made your point with reason and kindness, but not so long that the subject is over-thought. Don't procrastinate the end of the meeting.

You might also think about replacing no with not now or not yet. That leaves the door open for further communications, better ideas to come across which you might find perfect for your next project. Remember, a *no* to the project does not have to be a *no* to the worker.

You may also offer an alternative. Instead of no, perhaps the notion has inspired you to improve the idea. If you can encourage the person to investigate other venues as yet undiscovered and then come back for another meeting. It tables the problem and makes way for a better answer. That's an example of using procrastination in a positive way, as we've discussed.

But if you have to say no, that can be a real trauma for some people. They can hardly bring themselves to do it. For them, or perhaps you, here are some tips and tricks to make it easier to do.

Be direct about it. No need to beat around the bush. Just say, *"No, I can't,"* or *"That's not for me."* And there's no reason to put it off either, that's procrastination of the worst sort and it will only increase your anxiety. Face the moment when it happens.

Remember that there's no reason to apologize or make excuses. Excessive people-pleasing should be avoided, lest you be overly reliant upon their approval. We've seen the trouble that can cause!

Don't lie, either. There's no need to, and it will only increase your guilt. Not only did you back out of something and disappoint someone, but you've also lied about it! Who needs all that anxiety?

If you don't say *no* now, you may be resentful of being embroiled in an unwanted task later. Don't let that kind of passive/aggressive behavior spoil your life.

However, there's no reason not be polite. You can always toss in a friendly, *"Thanks for asking though."*

You might want to practice saying *no*. Pretend somebody is asking you do something when you're alone, and say *no*. Try it with a friend. Break the big task down into smaller tasks.

Above all, keep in mind that your self-worth is not related to how much you may do for others, but for what you do for yourself.

What if somebody doesn't take no for an answer? Be courteous but assertive and simply repeat your position. Set boundaries and stick to them. *No* still means *no*, after all. Or you might turn it back onto the other person. If they insist, ask them why or explore other options with them.

Want to have your mind blown? If you can't say *no*, remember that every *no* is a *yes* to something else. Turning down a work project may mean saying *yes* to avoiding a disaster, or *yes* to more time with family and friends. So, you're not really saying no at all. It's not a matter of rejection, but selection.

HOW TO CREATE A SIMPLE TO-DO LIST THAT MAKES BEING PRODUCTIVE EASY, INSTEAD OF LEAVING YOU FEELING ANXIOUS

To-do lists are a powerful tool for organization, motivation, and tackling procrastination and overthinking, among so many other habitually negative behaviors. But an overreliance on them can be dangerous. Often times the lists themselves can become unmanageable.

Make sure every action on the list is important enough to warrant your attention. Get rid of the low-value tasks and more pleasant tasks for later if you need to. Start with a new list for every day and think about doing a weekly version too. This will keep the daily lists shorter and more well-organized.

There are three techniques to creating a workable to-do list.

You may start every day by picking one to three important tasks you'll focus on that day and make them your highest priority.

Or, at the end of the workday, you may select up to six tasks for the next day, in order of highest priority. Then put that list into action the next day, making sure they all get done.

Or you may choose 13 tasks of different priorities; one high-priority, three medium- and nine low-priority tasks. Complete them in order of high priority to low.

Instead of a to-do list, you might make a might-do list, to lesser the pressure and account for unexpected interruptions and distractions. Some recommend three columns per list; *to-do, doing,* and *done.* The approach helps the worker chart progress and rewards small achievements and reinforces self-efficacy.

Some people recommend publishing your to-do list, which we know can add motivation to get that list done. Others recommend drawing the list to embed it into your brain and excite your attention, though that may be time consuming. You can always put it on your to-do list though!

Other tips for better to-do lists include doing them in color to encode priority; red for important, blue for low-value, and so on. Or you may give each task a pleasant name; project flowers, project puppy dogs. It may take a lot of the misery out of the task, and it'll certainly will make it less intimidating. Words have meaning.

As it is with everything these days, there are apps and websites to assist with your to-do list management, including *Minimalist, Google Tasks, A Text File, Slack,* and others.

MULTITASKING MAY SEEM A WISE MOVE AT FIRST, BUT NOT ALWAYS. KEEPING A TIGHT LEASH ON HOW YOU SPEND YOUR ENERGY

While to-do lists have all kinds of benefits, some suggest they represent a misdirection of focus. A lot of professionals suggest that, instead of managing time, one should be managing energy. There's more than enough time, they suggest, but energy fails and that's the weak link in the chain.

You have 24 hours every day, after all, but you don't bring the same energy to every day. As we've discussed, your energy level is heavily influenced by your sleep and eating habits, lack of reasonable breaks and burnout, who we are with and what we think about, how we move or don't and how much or how little, our emotions, and our purpose or the lack of one.

Researchers believe that your purpose is the driving force of your energy. The greater your purpose, the more energy you will be able to muster for it.

It's also true that habits can either waste time and energy or increase both. Surfing the internet is a habit which may waste time and energy but taking a walk will not only increase energy for all kinds of biological reasons, but the time invested in it will increase productivity once work resumes.

In Spain, a three-hour siesta during the hottest hours of the day is a tradition, but that won't work in today's United States or almost anywhere else. There's too much to do. And sleeping three hours a day could have adverse influences on the individual in any number of ways.

But there are components of the siesta which could be quite beneficial. Quick naps during the day can be refreshing, after all, and revitalize the body and brain. Scheduled breaks, which we already know are beneficial, should be observed. But breaks should come in moderation, like all things. Too many breaks lessen productivity and encourage the protagonist /overthinking cycle of shame and depression and, ultimately, inactivity.

Remember also that energy comes in different types and can be wasted or harvested in different ways. Emotional energy is rooted in feeling beyond reason, mental energy is rooted in feeling which is within the boundaries of reason and intellect, and spiritual energy is rooted in the feeling in the strength of some transcendental belief. If you can recognize which type of energy makes you strongest, you can prioritize behaviors which foster that kind of energy. If emotional energy saps you, you can know to avoid the triggers for that kind of energy. If mental energy is your strength, foster it with reading and writing and learning new skills. If spiritual energy is what sees you through, spend more time volunteering at your favored place of prayer.

With all we've discussed, it shouldn't be a surprise that food has a tremendous influence on a person's energy. Processed foods, those which are sugary, fatty, or salty, don't nourish the system, they exhaust it with a labored digestive process. Organic foods and those rich is vitamins, nutrients, and natural proteins fuel the body with more energy. If you're governing your energy intake and outgo, diet is the first place you should go.

Caffeine is both a famous and infamous source of energy. A cup of green tea may contain up to 25mg of caffeine, the same amount of black tea up to 42mg, while a cup of brewed coffee may contain up to or more than 108mg.

Studies show that coffee offers a stronger rush earlier on, but that inspires a deeper crash later, while the lesser amounts of caffeine in tea offer less of an initial boost but a more sustained energy level.

Six ways of getting more from caffeine, and losing less to it, include drinking coffee or tea less, but over longer periods of time. Consider taking breaks between cups of coffee or tea for the same result. Drink water with your coffee to cut the caffeine rush. Stay away from those energy drinks, as they're packed with caffeine and are likely to produce an intense energy rush and then a deep, hard crash, probably sooner rather than later.

Eat well and don't drink caffeine on an empty stomach. That's a bit counter-intuitive because a lot of people drink coffee first think in the morning, before they have an appetite or a chance to eat any food. Still, this can lead to digestive problems and anxiety.

Now that we've learned more about setting goals, let's take a closer look at developing new routines!

LET'S DEVELOP YOUR NEW ROUTINES

WHAT YOU SHOULD KNOW ABOUT HABITS

Okay, we've looked at a number of aspects of procrastination and overthinking, and a few other things as well, mostly focused on reversing these established, negative behaviors. And, as we've seen, it's easier to pick up a new habit than drop an old one, so if you're trying to correct an old behavior, simply pick up the habit of the opposite behavior.

But bad habits like overthinking and procrastination, clearly our focus here, have to be well understood before they can be effectively manipulated. And to best understand a thing, you have to get to its roots.

All habits are often born of the three Rs; reminder (the trigger which touches off feelings that inspire the negative behavior), routine (which is the negative behavior itself), and reward (the emotion generated by the behavior). A big meal (trigger) may make you want a cigarette, so you smoke one (routine) and enjoy that rush of nicotine (reward).

It's pretty easy to see that you could break this cycle at any point in the cycle. Change your triggers and eat only light meals. Some people graze, or simply eat little snacks through the day and don't have any big, traditional meals. Some experts believe this is a healthier way to eat. Or you could change your routine by chewing a piece of gum instead of smoking a cigarette, which is a common substitute. This changes the reward from a nicotine rush to a slight sugar buzz, perhaps. It's still a reward, right?

Identifying triggers can be helpful. Take note of when the reminders, or triggers, strike by noting when the routines, or behaviors, occur. Do you smoke more at night than during the day? Take a closer look at why. Are you generally alone, or are other people involved? Is there one thing in particular which seems to inspire the desire to smoke? You'll find your triggers lurking in one of these questions. That'll help you root them out and either change or avoid them.

When changing your habits and developing new routines, keep in mind your inspiration for it, your long-term goal. That will give you motivation to carry on through the many smaller tasks which will be necessary to get the big task done.

And you can use the same techniques you've already started to develop! Enlist a friend for support and to be a sounding board, allowing you to vocalize your goals and give you advice you may need. Be mindful of what you're doing at all times, so you don't slip into old habits. Know what you're doing and why. Replace one habit with the opposite habit.

BREAKING BAD AND UNHEALTHY HABITS

What causes bad habits in the first place? Knowing the cause will help you discover the cure. As we often say, the answer is usually sitting right next to the question (or in this case, the solution is right next to the problem).

One aspect to the continuation of bad habits is the so-called *loophole*. Think of the loophole as the justification for the behavior. Being stressed out justifies the need for a calming cigarette break. Being bored often justifies overeating.

Now that you know what a loophole is, let's take a look at the different varieties of this insidious part of the bad-habit cycle.

First, there's the *false choice* loophole, where there's always something else to get done, It's a very common loophole. There's also the *moral licensing* loophole, where good behavior rationalizes the reward of bad behavior.

The *tomorrow loophole* is procrastination incarnate, putting off until tomorrow what could just as easily be done today. The *lack of control* loophole is the gambit of helplessness and submission to the bad behavior.

You may employ the *planning to fail* loophole, when you assume what you will try is doomed to failure and is unworthy of the effort.

The *This doesn't count* loophole provides convenient excuses like sickness or vacation to avoid the task.

The *one-coin* loophole assures us that there's always another chance, another day.

There's also the *questionable assumption* loophole, doubting the reason for the act; the *concern for others* loophole puts the blame on possible adverse reactions of or damage to others. The *fake self-actualization* loophole may convince you that there's no time to work toward long-term goals, that you must live only in the moment. This, of course, is a bastardization of the Buddhist notion of abandoning living in the past or future and to embrace the moment. The difference is in the grounding of the belief. For some, it's wisdom. For others, it's an excuse. If a Buddhist monk says this to you, give it some thought. If the person knows nothing of Buddhism or meditation and simply parrots the line, it's just an excuse.

There's also a biological aspect to bad habits.

The limbic system, the emotional parts of the human brain holds onto habits, as they are automated and easier to perform. But the prefrontal cortex controls the more disciplined activities. So, look to the limbic system as the root of your procrastination. Experts consider the limbic to be the older part of the brain and the prefrontal cortex the newer. Of course, all parts of a single brain are the same age. But emotional parts evolved first as a matter of evolutionary fact. Emotion secured survival and, slowly reason and discipline began to evolve based on the emotional core that was already there. Think about the discovery of fire, the domestication of animals, the change of prehistoric lifestyle from monadism to establishing fixed communities, or clans. We were emotional first, and we still do tend to put emotions first because that part of the brain has been developing over a longer period of time.

Stress and boredom are the root of a lot of bad habits. We're looking for an amusement to counter the difficult or tedious parts of our lives, and those are crucial in the procrastination and overthinking cycle. So, while it's difficult to avoid these triggers, or reminders, you can always change your routine. If distractions are a common respite from boredom, take a walk instead. It has every benefit of health and mind which watching YouTube videos of dancing cats simply doesn't. Conversely, we've already seen the detriment of spending too much time in one place. If you're not working, why use your workstation for amusements? Change your environment, a practice you should recognize by now as being amazingly impactful on any frame of mind.

Another well-used technique is to visualize. Imagine yourself not having to rush out for cigarettes first thing in the morning. Visualize yourself warm inside with your family and friends while others stand out in the cold smoking their cigarettes in isolation.

And don't personalize it. You're not your habits; you can always improve.

And there are a few concrete steps and exercises which will help you break just about any bad or unhealthy habit.

You might consider leaving yourself Post-it notes to remind you to curb a certain routine. If your long-term goal is to go to Paris, but you want to lose 20 pounds first, just write *Paris* on a Post-it and stick it on the refrigerator door.

Just as we used *if/then* to moderate and modify our goals, try *but* here. You may smoke, *but* you're going to quit smoking. Don't just accept that being a smoker is part of who you are, like your height or your skin color.

We've seen the value of time tracking, and that's of value here too. When you feel the reminder, or trigger, or when you indulge in the routine, or behavior, write it town. Be detailed, not vague. Note the exact time, place, who you're with, what is happening. Then examine your log and note the patterns. The triggers will rise to the surface by appearing more commonly on your log.

THE POWER OF HEALTHY HABITS WILL HELP YOU CONQUER YOUR OVERTHINKING AND PROCRASTINATION

We've talked about replacing one habit with its opposite. And what are the opposite of bad habits? Good habits, of course, healthy habits instead of unhealthy habits. Some of those unhealthy habits include drinking too little water, eating too late at night, getting too little exercise and/or sleep. Eating too much sodium is another unhealthy habit, as is eating processed foods. A lot of times, so-called *fat-free* foods are worse than natural foods with natural fats.

Eating lunch at your desk and using too much olive oil are common unhealthy habits. Skipping dessert is also less healthy than it sounds, and keeping an unclean kitchen has lots of hidden health risks.

And these are all easy to correct. Keep your counters clean, have a piece of cake, stay away from any food that comes in a colorful box or plastic wrapper. Don't eat after eight pm. If you can do those few things, you can counter a number of common unhealthy habits.

You may not have heard of the *two-minute rule*, but it tells us that any new habit should only take about two minutes to do. This approach basically breaks down any task to its first, simplest step. Reading at night becomes reading a single page. Thirty minutes of yoga becomes simply pulling out the yoga mat. The habit of studying for class becomes simply opening the books and leaving them open. Running three miles becomes a walk around the block.

It's another way of breaking down the big task into smaller, manageable tasks with concrete goals, the rewards of which propel further performance. Naturally, this is a stepping-stone technique! Stopping at two minutes of anything won't get you far.

This micro-habit technique is popular with a lot of experts, who also assert that there are habits that most successful people share. These are the healthy habits you can adopt to counter the negative ones.

Practice passion do what you love even if you don't do it professionally and do it passionately. Read and workout to keep your mind and body strong and clean. Save money. Have a mentor and be a mentor. Be mindful of relationships and of selfcare. Work even when you're not inspired and quiet the so-called monkey brain, that part which is so easily distracted. Do this by using a mantra. Donate time and money to inspire the feeling of self-efficacy. We've touched on all of these in this book, so it's remarkable to note that the world's great corporate successes employ them. And you can too!

Here's another helpful way to break old, negative habits and picking up new, healthy habits that will stick. First, make the old habit invisible, remove all cues. Then make it unattractive, remind yourself of all the negative aspects. Make it difficult, physically inconvenient. Make it unsatisfying, visualize the negative results and the immediate unpleasant consequences.

To make good habits stick, do basically the opposite. Make the healthy habit obvious instead of invisible. Make it attractive by visualizing the benefits of the healthy habit. Make it easy instead of difficult, make in convenient. Then make it satisfying by visualizing all the benefits and positive results and the immediate pleasurable rewards.

Apply cigarette smoking versus gum chewing and see how easily it works! Go ahead, I'll wait.

See? And it works every time, as do most of these techniques.

DAILY MEDITATION & MINDFULNESS CAN REVOLUTIONIZE YOUR MOMENT-BY-MOMENT HAPPINESS

Daily meditation and mindfulness are powerful techniques for creating healthy habits and they're both very healthy habits on their own. Meditation may help you better understand your mental and physical pain, help you connect better to yourself and others, lower stress and improve focus, and reduce negative self-talk and the easily distracted monkey brain.

Health benefits associated with meditation include lowered blood pressure and improved blood circulation, a lower heart rate and slower respiratory rate, reduced anxiety, stress, and perspiration, lower blood cortisol levels, a heightened sense of well-being and deeper relaxation.

Meditation has great calming effects. Research has shown that EEG activity actually decreases during meditation. Meditation also helps you to recharge so you have more energy throughout the day.

Meditation increases blood flow in the brain and may have positive neurological effects. It can also reduce the need for sleep. Meditation may slow the aging of the brain and enhance muscle control, emotions, and the senses of seeing, hearing, and the ability of speech.

Meditation helps achieve flow, or being *in the zone*. That, in turn, helps get more done and defeats procrastination. Medication has been proven to increase students' test scores up to eleven percent.

There are volumes on the shelves of our local bookstore about it, or on Amazon, but let's take a look at these practices as they relate to bad habits, goal setting, procrastination, and especially overthinking.

There is a variety of different meditation styles, each with its own benefits.

But first, how do you learn to meditate? In mindfulness meditation, we're learning how to pay attention to the breath as it goes in and out and notice when the mind wanders from this task. *Returning to the breath* strengthens your ability to be mindful and to pay attention and remain focused.

Meditation may provide space in your mind and in your life, and that's what the overthinker needs most. All you need to start is a comfortable place to sit, some patience, and some self-compassion (sometimes the hardest part).

But be prepared! Meditating may make you sleepy, and it may be hard to find the time. It's well worth it though!

Paying attention to your breath teaches you to return to and remain in the present moment, abandoning the past and the future. That's what the overthinker needs most.

In mindful meditation, you pay attention to each breath and concentrate on only that. In and out, the natural connection of inside and outside. Keep focusing on it as you do it, don't let your mind wander. Fix on the simple, natural, nurturing act of breathing.

How do you learn to meditate? In mindfulness meditation, we're learning how to pay attention to the breath as it goes in and out, and notice when the mind wanders from this task. This practice of returning to the breath builds the muscles of attention and mindfulness.

It's that simple, but it does require practice. The more you do it, the better you'll be and the better the results will be.

To practice this powerful technique, first sit down and get comfortable. Prepare yourself to be sitting still for the next few minutes. Set a time limit, especially when you start. Like all things, break the big task down into manageable smaller tasks.

Now focus on your breath. Where is it going inside you? Are you filling your lungs or just your nose? Is your breathing regular? Do this for about two minutes, then inhale and exhale deeply and slowly.

Repeat this cycle for as long as you can, and you'll note the amazing benefits. You can vary the cycle too, using a fixed focal point to focus on instead of breathing.

Mindfulness is a word we've been using a lot, and it deserves a closer look. Mindfulness is that consciousness of behavior which we so often overlook. Bathing, eating, driving, social interaction, even work, become collections of automated behavior that we just don't think about. Breathing is one of these; it's automatic, you don't have to concentrate on it in order to make it happen.

But a lack of mindfulness creates sloppy work, bad health habits, careless or reckless driving, failed relationships, because we just don't think about what we're doing. We're repeating the same things we've done for years, and in pretty much the same way.

Ways to be mindful are easy to apply! Practice mindfulness during routine activities like sweeping or cooking. Practice mindfulness first thing in the morning for a mindful start to the day. But don't restrict your mind from wandering, that's part of the exercise. You'll become skilled at bringing yourself back into the focus of mindfulness.

But keep it short. You don't want to stretch yourself too thin with this exercise and be mindful of every little thing. One thing a day to start.

Practice mindfulness while you wait; long lines and traffic are great times to refocus. You may want to pick a place or time, such as your coffee break, to practice mindfulness.

So, it takes a deliberate decision to be mindful of these things, of all things if you can be. Meditation uses mindfulness to guide focus. Mindfulness of something as basic and automatic as breathing is the perfect way to sharpen the skill of being mindful, strengthening the mindfulness muscle, which we can then use to greater effect in other aspects of our lives.

Body scan meditation is a simple and powerful technique too, which can be combined with any mindful meditation regiment. Just sit down where you are comfortable and sit quietly. Instead of focusing on your breath, or a single focal point, you'll be focusing on your body. Start with your feet and just feel them (not with your hands). Feel the blood running through them, the bones and tendons and muscles. Now scan upward through your legs, surveying their condition, feeling them as a part of your body. Progress upward through every part of your body to the top of your head It's a way of reconnecting with yourself, of becoming more comfortable in your own skin.

Walking meditation is another way to strengthen mindfulness. You don't have to be sitting down. You may focus on counting your steps, up to 10 then back again. The important thing is to fix on something simple, to clear your mind and not clutter it. And given all the health and mental benefits of walking, this is a beneficial technique in several ways. Do watch where you're walking, however!

Loving-kindness meditation has its own challenges for perfectionist protagonists and negative self-talkers as it relies on self-compassion, hard for some to achieve. Loving-kindness meditation focuses on the positivity of the person meditating, on their lives. It celebrates good-heartedness and open-mindedness and forgiveness.

Try using a mantra to practice loving kindness, such as, *"May I live in safety", "May I have peace, joy," "May I live with ease," "May I have physical happiness* (or health, or freedom from pain, depending on your needs)."

Spiritual meditation allows you to focus, not on your body or your breath or on a fixed focal point, but on God or whatever is the source of the mediator's spiritual faith. The goal is to be closer to oneself by being closer to god. Potent oils and incenses are often used, such as frankincense and myrrh, sage and cedar, sandalwood and palo santo.

Focused meditation focuses on other things; counting beads, a song. Mantra meditation uses a simple monotone to focus on, like the famous, *"Oooouummmmmmmm ..."*

Transcendental meditation is perhaps the most well-known. It builds on mantra meditation but includes more sophisticated mantras specific to the reader.

In Visualization meditation the meditator imagines themselves at that place where the goal is achieved, visualize what that will look like, focus on that.

You may have questions about meditation. If you do, you're certainly not alone! Here are a few commonly asked questions about meditation and, of course, their answers.

Q) What if I have an itch?
A) Resist it if you can, try to scratch it with your mind. Failing that, scratch it. You're trying to focus on other things, and an itch is a terrible distraction and one that's easy to deal with.

Q) Should my breath be slow or fast or regular?
A) Just relax and breathe. A natural breathing rate will find itself, most likely. Breathe too fast and you may pass out!

Q) Should I close my eyes?
A) If you like, but it won't make using a focal point much easier! It could make walking therapy absolutely hazardous. A lot of people do close their eyes during mindful meditation, yes. If you do, take it easy. There's no reason to clamp them shut. Make it easy.

Q) Maybe I just can't do this?
A) Everybody thinks that, and it doesn't stop them. It shouldn't stop you. You *can* do this, but it will take practice. Remember that nothing worth doing is ever easy.

Q) Should I meditate alone or in a group?
A) Either, depending on your preference. Consider both!

Q) Is there an optimal time of day to meditate?

A) Not really, as long as it remains convenient, but tomorrow doesn't count!

Q) What should I do if I become aroused?

A) Accept that your mind will wander and just bring yourself back to your point of focus. No worries.

Q) Should I involve my pet?

A) As long as you don't interact with your pet, it's fine for them to sit quietly with you.

Q) How long should I meditate for?

A) It's more about regularity than duration. As long as you do it every day, it can be for as little as five minutes. Make it convenient and attractive.

Q) What should I wear?

A) Something comfortable.

DON'T BECOME A SLAVE TO TECHNOLOGY, YOU SHOULD BE THE MASTER OF IT

Truly, information is at the heart of the technological age. But some information is useful, some merely entertaining. Generally, the more entertaining a certain piece of information is, the less useful it's likely to be.

Either way, technology is everywhere in our modern world, and it is one of the most potent sources of distraction and brain clutter there could ever be, fostering monkey brain and triggering all manner of behaviors. But we do need our phones and computers and the internet just to survive. Banking, remote working, connecting with family and friends, technology is at the heart of our lives and that's not likely to change anytime soon.

There are lots of benefits to reducing your tech time. Studies show that computer light can be harmful to the eyes, posture can be adversely affected. Staring at your phone prevents you from fully interacting with others, leading to missed opportunities. Time spent playing app games on a smartphone could be better spent daydreaming or meditating or conjuring up new goals to set and tasks to achieve. It encourages rudeness when a person meets with another and then spends the whole time on the phone with somebody else. That's always been considered discourteous even in the time of land-lines. And the internet is rife with all kinds of misinformation and dangerous people who could easily victimize the unwary internet surfer.

So how can you prevent yourself from becoming a slave to all this tech?

With streaming sites like Netflix, so-called *binge watching* has become a trend. But that doesn't mean you have to sit in front of the TV or computer. Clean, cook, sew, do laundry, work out; there are all manner of useful chores can get done while the Trailer Park Boys are up to their goofy hijinks.

If you feel yourself overwhelmed by too much information, go back to our established tips and tricks. Write down everything you watch and categorize it, ranking it by quality on a scale of one to ten. Then eliminate the bottom 20%. Or, if that's too drastic, pick three things of the bottom 20% and temporarily replace them with something else. You can always switch back.

Say no to three things this week, it almost doesn't matter what they are. As long as you're eliminating these tech-oriented distractions for this week and see how you feel about it next week. Include all this in your log or make a new one just for this experiment.

Some people are visual learners, some learn better from hearing things. Know which you are and emphasize these things in your tech time. Visual learners may prefer to read a book, audio-oriented learners might spend more time with an audiobook.

Cut back on the quantity of all your tech time. Log up your time on phone, computer, iPod, and tablet, and reduce all by 10%. It's an uncomplicated way to reduce your use of, and dependence on, high tech. You can spend that time meditating, walking, visiting with friends, or enjoying a healthy, nourishing meal.

Some researchers, individuals, and families have adopted a new protocol for dealing with the intrusiveness of high tech on their lives, the new etiquette of the digital era:

No phones during mealtimes, social gatherings, or driving. No high tech for kids under a certain age. No phones as music players; use an mp3 or other dedicated music player. No high tech in the bedroom, or strict time limits. No ring-tone notifications. Those are for phone calls. No smart watches unless it is for health-oriented purposes. No phone app notifications. Keep two computers, one for work and one for play. Keep the play computer out of sight until appropriate.

Now that we've got a better grip on managing our energy and our tech, let's take a closer look not just at managing time, but using it wisely... hopefully without too much high tech!

TIME MANAGEMENT IS THE ANSWER TO MOST OF YOUR PROBLEMS

Time management is at the heart of what procrastinators and over-thinkers suffer from and seek to overcome. While it's true that energy is important to manage on its own, time management remains essential. And the tips and tricks to help become a better time manager are the same as the others. It's amazing how this relatively simple set of skills can be applied to so many levels of the same challenges, and to different challenges altogether.

Time management has amazing benefits. You'll get better results, faster. You'll be more productive. You'll waste less time and avoid complications and conflicts. Better time management helps clear your slate for leisure time, which is good for a balanced life. That makes you calmer and gives you more opportunities to avoid stress. In the workplace, you won't miss deadlines or be late for appointments, your focus will be more fixed, you'll avoid stress. You'll avoid penalties for failure and enjoy greater rewards for your success.

Time management encourages patience, focus, organizational skills, decision-making, plan-making, motivation, goal setting and self-awareness.

So, as we approach other challenges, we look at time management as something which can be handled in (hopefully) recognizable steps. It begins with effective planning and is followed by setting the right goals and objectives. Reasonable deadlines and delegation of responsibilities (in a team setting) before prioritizing tasks in order of importance and then allocating the proper amount of time to that activity.

In general, use what you've learned to be a better time manager. Make lists and time logs, prioritize tasks, set the right goals and so on. Be selective and abandon perfectionism. Focus on the task, not yourself.

But what if you're a shift worker or have some other job which makes time management even more difficult? Let's take a look.

You may not have heard of the 80/20 rule. It holds that 20% of our efforts wind up resulting in 80% of our outcomes.

LEARN TO PRIORITIZE WHAT YOU'LL DO NEXT

Prioritizing is a big part of getting things done, as we've already seen. So, let's take a closer look at how to best prioritize our tasks. You may recall the matrix we used about priority, that there are urgent tasks and important tasks. Important tasks are more closely associated with long-term goals, and urgent tasks are more short-term. Some are important but not urgent, some urgent but not important. Use the matrix help prioritize your tasks, as we've seen. It's just another example of how these principles operate across the board. Master them, and you can apply them to every level of everything in your life.

We've been talking about breaking things down into smaller parts, and (hopefully) it's worked. But there's another way to look at it, especially if you're prioritizing. You might want to gather your smaller to-do lists into one big master task list. This will help you see them all in a single context and you'll be able to prioritize each list. That's what prioritization is all about, right?

There's a funny turn of phrase, *eat the frog*. Attributed to Mark Twain, who said something like, "If your job is to eat a frog, it's best to do it first thing in the morning." It's a beautiful illustration of prioritization. Get the biggest, most unpleasant job done first, it'll make everything else seem easy as pie … which is a lot tastier than frog!

Some people prioritize by alphabetic notation. The so-called *ABCDE method* rates tasks in that order of priority. It may work for you.

Now let's move into the third section of this book and continue to look outward, rather than inward. Our next subject, your support partner!

III

IMPLEMENTATION

FINDING AN ACCOUNTABILITY PARTNER COULD SUPERCHARGE YOUR SUCCESS

WHY AN ACCOUNTABILITY PARTNER CAN MAKE THE CHANGE THAT YOU ARE HOPING TO HAVE IN YOUR LIFE

We've already looked at the many benefits of having a support partner. They can provide advice and compassion, a sounding board and a commitment board. They can impart good advice, help you reason out bad ideas, set goals, change self-efficacy. A support or accountability partner is invaluable.

Think of all the successful institutional pairings in history; any US president and his vice-president, any golfer and his caddie, any boxer and his coach, any superhero and his sidekick. Scuba divers go down using the buddy system. Most incredible of all, people are still getting married! The buddy partner works, but ... why?

They curb procrastination and urge a mentee to stay on track. Once that behavior is learned, it inevitably takes hold. Support partners keep you motivated and help ensure you meet your goals. They offer a different, more enlightened perspective, and can positively influence goal-setting and other crucial steps. And, as accountability partners, they hold you accountable if you falter and to stick to your deadlines. A lot of people need that support, and they should have it … and they can get it!

THE CHOOSING PHASE, THE QUALITIES OF AN ACCOUNTABILITY PARTNER THAT YOU SHOULD SEEK

How do you best find or choose an accountability partner? It may not be as easy as it seems. Some in your line of work may be too competitive, or fear giving up their secrets. Others may be too busy or just too selfish. Some aren't cut out to be mentors either.

First of all, make sure you choose your accountability partner based on your goals. If you want to succeed in advertising, look for somebody who knows the field. A Catholic priest may not be the best choice. If you're putting a corporate team together, you might seek out a high school football coach, or somebody skilled in team-building who might bring a new and competitive voice to your efforts.

Once you know what you're looking to do and who might be best to help, ask your friends if they know anybody who might be interested in helping. Coaches love to coach; teachers love to teach. Consider a professor at your local university who specializes in the field you're pursuing.

Joining classes is a great way to find an accountability partner. The gym is a good way too or volunteering at any number of places eager for some extra help. There you'll find people ready and willing to share their time and influence, just like you are. If you were working at a food bank and some young person asked for your support, you'd give it, right? Right.

And these days, you can find the support you need online. Whatever you're doing or whatever subjects your project may touch upon, there's a Facebook group or an online forum about it. That is an invaluable resource for finding not just one support group but dozens, and from all around the world! There's never been a better time to be supported by people in this way. Beware of trolls, of course.

There are even apps like *Fitstream* to help build support and account-ability groups.

One part of the process of choosing an accountability partner, of course, is being one. Having a mentor and mentoring someone else is still key to our regiment, up and down the board. Each has its distinct benefits.

And for the stage in life when you want to mentor, consider what it takes to be a good support partner.

You'll have to be supportive. Sure, you'll start off with that impulse, it's at the heart of what you're doing. Still, you're not there to be a contrarian, to play the devil's advocate. Support means support.

You'll want to focus on the goal, not the person. Always depersonalize these things.

You'll want to prioritize listening and understanding. Don't just nod and smile but invest yourself in these challenges and draw upon your experience to be a truly valuable resource. That's why you're doing it, after all.

You'll want to keep the lines of communications open in both directions. And when you communicate, be thoughtful in your counsel. Your mentee will be listening and just may follow our advice, so be careful what you say and how you say it. They may personalize your advice, especially if it's critical of the work.

Once you commit to a mentorship, don't quit. They may quit you, but if you abandon the mentee that could trigger feelings of failure, of anger, and could begin the procrastination or overthinking cycles which we're all here to suppress.

And be open to sharing your life. That's where your greatest wisdom is, after all. And it will help build trust and make you a better mentor.

HOW TO TACKLE THE BIGGEST & MOST IMPORTANT PROJECTS THAT WE ALL LOVE TO PROCRASTINATE ON

CHANGE COMES WITHIN AND YOU MUST CHOOSE IT YOURSELF

E lizabeth Kubler-Ross created the change curve looking at how people dealt with a terminal diagnosis. It measures confidence and morale against looking to the past and looking to the future. The four stages of the curve are information, support, direction, and encouragement. Interestingly, they correlate to the five stages of grief: Denial, anger, bargaining, depression, acceptance.

It sounds a bit complicated, but it works something like this: In stage one of the curve, information. When the diagnosis comes, the patient is apt to suffer a loss of a high degree of confidence and experience denial. The second stage lends support to the patient, though confidence and morale are likely to plummet and anger more likely to rise. The third stage of the curve, direction, tends to raise the patient's confidence and morale as they explore new options. Stage four of the curve, encouragement, tends to boost both morale and acceptance.

The model can be helpful, not only with a terminal diagnosis, but any change. Divorce, news of pregnancy, the end of a romance, a job loss or even a job promotion! When change comes to you, think about these stages and understand what stage you're in and how you're reacting to it emotionally. Understanding these things will help you to control them, in fact it's the only way to control them. Knowledge is power!

There's an old saying which was made very popular in Alcoholics Anonymous, and it's known as the *serenity prayer*:

God, grant me the serenity to accept the things I cannot change, the courage to change the things I can, and the wisdom to know the difference.

And it's effective for all kinds of change when that change is hard to deal with. But let's look at this time-worn bit of wisdom a bit more closely to see how we can apply it to our personal and professional lives.

When you're managing personal change, it is vital to accept the things you cannot change. Think of the overthinker, who constantly replays bygone disagreements, saying in their minds what they didn't say at the time, wondering what might have been said to create a different outcome. But that cannot be changed. The past has passed. So, it's a waste of time and creates all manner of negative behaviors. In looking ahead to manage your own personal change, keep this part of the serenity prayer in mind too. You'll never be taller; you'll never regrow that hair. Don't even waste your time trying. Instead, focus your time on the next part of the prayer.

If there are things you *can* change, then make a plan to change them. If a degree would increase your chances of success, make a plan to earn one. That big task would include just about every technique we've discussed in this book, but that would be a thing you could change. First, you'd need a plan. Losing weight, quitting smoking, getting control of your temper; all of these can be changed, but they need a plan which includes small goals leading to the ultimate goal, a timetable, and other analytical steps as we've already discussed.

Knowing the difference is what stops the overthinker, as the things which can't be changed are often perceived as if they could be. Future events can be affected by what we do in the present, right? Some of them can be, yes. Then again ... you control your finances, but not the overall economy. As too many people learned, you can do everything right in preparing for your future, but economic forces may undo your years of diligence. You can control how much you spend or save, but you can't control a recession.

But you can be a strategic thinker and prepare for contingencies. We talked earlier about including time for complexities which arise suddenly, and when you're managing your own change and your own future, give yourself a margin for the unexpected, and then be prepared to accept it when it happens.

Abraham H. Maslow, famous for his *hierarchy of needs*, once said, "One can choose to go back toward safety or forward toward growth.

Growth must be chosen again and again; fear must be overcome again and again."

It's clear how this applies to managing your own change. Personal growth and change don't just happen, and if they do, they become twisted and unruly. You (or anyone) must take control of that growth and change, shape it properly, manage it constantly. Also, personal growth is not a one-and-done deal, it's a process. So be prepared to embark on a long journey. If you're not prepared, you're likely to backslide. It happens to a lot of people who mistake the first step for the entire journey.

Or you may think of personal growth as a savings account which only grows as you contribute to it over time.

Personal growth, in fact one could say that the person you are, is defined by the choices made. Better choices make for more personal growth which makes a better person. And, as almost always, there is a cyclical nature to this construct. The lesser choices make for less or no personal growth which makes a lesser person who makes even lesser choices which make for even less or no personal growth which make an even lesser person who makes further lesser choices and so on. The cycle feeds itself and the spiral either goes up or down. Which direction it goes is up to you.

So, when you're making these choices which will drive your personal growth up or down, you may ask yourself, *"Am I going to regret this choice? Is this in line with my integrity and my values? What will I gain from this and what will I lose?"*

You'll know what the answers are. It's just that most people don't ask the questions before they act or react. It's always wise to step back and consider before any action is taken. That's a technique we learned from active procrastination, which is actually a positive behavior.

SHOULD YOU RELY ON YOUR IMPLICIT MEMORY, YES OR NO?

Implicit memory can be described as engrained, automated into your behavior. One of its subsets is procedural memory. Tying your shoes or riding a bike are capabilities stored in your procedural memory. Implicit memory is a higher grade of this kind of memory, often called unconscious or automatic memory. Athletes, dancers, and musicians know it as *muscle memory.* Years of repetition make certain functions, like throwing a football or playing a musical chord, virtually automatic. Recalling words to a song is another example or driving a car.

There is also explicit memory, wherein a conscious effort is made to retrieve memories. Thoughts of historical facts, events on a vacation, people you knew all reside in your explicit memory. Unlike implicit memories, explicit memories are vulnerable to loss.

And there are two types of explicit memories. There are memories of specific events, like your wedding day or what you did last week; these are episodic memories. Semantic memories include names, dates, historical facts, general knowledge which is not so particular to episodes in your life. Episodic and semantic memories, the two subsets of explicit memory.

Research shows that stress and mood have a strong influence on the formation of both semantic and episodic memories, and so does age. It's pretty well-known that both types of explicit memories fade with time and the effects of aging on the brain. But it's also true that semantic memories may become unreliable as well. They're still more reliable than explicit memories, but our faith in them as being just about 100% may not be as accurate as we thought.

But there are ways to test implicit memory. Researchers have three ways to measure the loss of this essential function.

In the word stem completion test, the subject is given several alphabetic letters and instructed to provide a word which starts which each of those letters. Seems fairly easy, right? Try it now: A, C, E, O. I'll wait. Okay, while you did yours, I came up with *apple, chalk, example, owl.*

In the word fragment test, the subject is presented with an incomplete word and asked to complete it, such as *restaura__, bycic__, free_ay, au_omob_le,* and so on. If you squint your eyes, you can see the complete word based on your implicit memory of those words.

There's also the anagram solving test, where the subject is given a jumble and instructed to rearrange them in the proper order: *takecj (jacket), repnosltaiy, (personality).* That last one would make a good game show!

There are also different types of implicit memory.

Procedural memory, which we've already touched on, includes learned behaviors which become automatic, tying your shoes or riding a bike.

But there's also *priming*, wherein reactions become automatic. How many people were afraid to go into the water after JAWS? That was because the movie primed them to be fearful of sharks. There's also classical conditioning, which trains the subject to automatically respond to a certain stimulus, like Pavlov's dog. If you don't know, Pavlov rang a bell and gave his dog a treat. He did it repeatedly, so that the dog was conditioned to anticipate the treat when the bell rang. Then he rang the bell and didn't give the dog a treat, and the dog waited patiently for the treat.

Implicit memory is a kind of long-term memory, and long-term memories have a big impact on your activities and behaviors. They're formative.

Short-term memories, on the other hand, last for less than a minute. They may become long-term memories with some effort (the name of someone you just met) unless they're absolutely spectacular (a first kiss).

ESTABLISH YOUR SELF-DISCIPLINE AND SELF-CONTROL, AND DON'T LET ANYTHING HINDER YOU FROM WHAT YOU MUST DO

Finding motivation is a crucial step in establishing and developing your self-discipline. You may be motivated by life's necessities, such as feeding yourself or your family or obtaining safe or better shelter. You may want to help others, once you've seen to your own hierarchy of needs. You may want to achieve something that will transcend you and speak to others whom you will never know. You may simply want to have a happier life, to enjoy yourself more.

Here are a few questions to guide your decisions to apply reason to your desire and increase your self-discipline. Make a list (naturally) of what things you want and how many. Are they reasonable things? Are the amounts reasonable? Maybe you can cut the amount in half. Would that rob your life of its joy? Would your head explode?

Ask yourself again how much you want the object. Would you commit a crime to get it? What would you sacrifice to have that thing? How much do you want the object? How much joy do you get, or will you get from the object? Is it worth the inherent risk? How much will it hurt not to have it?

Answering these questions will help you establish and improve your self-discipline and that will help with everything else you do. Don't wait for it be resultant of your other efforts, make it the wellspring of the other campaigns. They'll work together, but self-discipline really is a good place to start.

Are you lacking in self-discipline? Do you have overwhelming desires to do something you know is bad for you? Do you succumb to those desires? How often? Are you disgusted at the idea of doing something which may be good for you? How often do you succumb to this disgust and fail to do the task? The answer will tell you.

Let's try a little experiment. Think of something you really want; a drink, a cigarette, your favorite food, a new car.

Now rate it on a scale from 1 to 10 based on these questions: *"How much do I want it? How disappointed will I be if I don't get it? Do I want it, or do I need it, do I really have to have it?"*

Consider how pained you will be if you don't do or get what you're considering. Rate on the scale the statements, *"I have to have a cigarette. I didn't have one yesterday and it ruined my day. I haven't had one for two days, maybe I can wait until tomorrow."*

Once again, we see that the tried-and-true techniques we've used before will work perfectly here. Establishing self-discipline is, after all, a large task which you'll want to break up into smaller tasks, each with a timeline. You'll want to log your activities and progress, state your intentions and get a support partner and so on. Focus, persistence, organization, resilience, responsibility, and a strong work ethic are all traits of people who practice self-discipline.

Self-discipline, like those other traits, are learned behaviors and they are forged in time and experience. And it has its own inherent challenges. If you know these challenges, you'll be better equipped to handle them when they come along.

The road to self-discipline will challenge your perceptions, for instance. It's the old bugaboo of self-efficacy. Some people just don't believe that they can be more disciplined. They are who they are. We've seen this pop in several different ways throughout our studies so far. But it may be particularly challenging when it comes to self-discipline. Why is that? Perhaps because self-discipline goes deeper than almost anything else we've touched on yet. Without self-discipline, all the goal setting and time-logging in the world won't come to much. It may, over time, sharpen one's self-discipline, of course. The methods we discussed are time-tested and laboratory-proven to help defeat procrastination and overthinking, and both of those are rife with a lack of self-discipline. Practicing them will naturally increase your self-discipline as a result.

But what if we turned it around, and put self-discipline where it belongs; as a cause or motivating factor instead of a symptom or a result? We'd see that this is the source of our strengths and our weaknesses. Those who have more self-discipline are better equipped to curb unhealthy behavior, after all.

Some people are lucky enough to have been raised in a strictly regulated home. I don't mean an abusive home, but it's known that children brought up under less supervision and less parental guidance get into more trouble. Kids with a more stable home fare better. Kids who play team sports are recorded as being more prosperous as adults. Why? Discipline is instilled in you in a more stable household or on a sports team.

But not everybody had that kind of upbringing. Some had working parents and were so-called *latch-key* kids. Some kids were loners and not athletic. I was in both categories. And a lot of people who weren't strictly disciplined as kids simply lack self-discipline as adults.

Those who have some self-discipline can always have more, and those who have less need more. Those who have none truly need it. The good news is that it can be learned, and at any time of life.

Some people may tell you that the first seven years of life are the formative years, where the basics of the individual are set. And to a degree, that's probably right. But people don't stop growing at seven years old. They evolve and change and become better people with greater depth. So, it's a fallacy to say that a person has no control over their self-discipline as a result of childhood experiences. It's entirely a personal choice.

So, how do you nurture self-motivation? Really, it brings us back to the set of skills we apply to just about everything. Find your motivation, set your goals, do a time log, get support, delegate if possible, abandon the mental stumbling blocks, practice self-sympathy.

Another way of getting around the challenges of self-discipline is to find a motivational activity. Think of this as the reward you'll get at the end of every small task. This time let it be something like watching an episode of your favorite TV show uninterrupted, or a long, hot bath.

An interesting thing about the quest for self-discipline, as with the other pursuits which should follow it and come before, is that you must become comfortable with failure. Perfectionism is a central challenge of procrastination and overthinking, but those are fueled by self-discipline. If perfectionism infects you at that root level, you may never get anywhere. In your quest for self-discipline, you'll fail several times, perhaps quite often. That's to be expected. Don't let the perfect be the enemy of the good. A fifty-percent success rate, and that's a failure for every success, is awesome. It will increase your self-discipline considerably. If you succeed only three times out of then, you'll hit 50% the next year, and incrementally increase year after year. Accept failure as a necessary part of the process.

HERE ARE A FEW TIPS AND TRICKS TO DEVELOP YOUR SELF-DISCIPLINE:

- Make it a habit by doing it once a day. Pick one thing to deny yourself, to press yourself to do. Just one thing a day, you can do it again the next day if you like, but deny yourself something else. It might be a treat, it might be a margin of tardiness, it might be leaving mail unopened. Sacrifice one of these every day. Not only will you strengthen your self-discipline, you'll actually be getting things done.

- Focus on one facet of your self-discipline at a time. This is a manner of breaking the big task into little tasks, like the previous exercise. But this will also keep you focused on that particular discipline. Distractions and multi-tasking will be especially detrimental here. This week, you'll get the place thoroughly cleaned. Next week, you can organize. The week after that, start getting into shape. You'll never be able to get all that done at once.

- Meditate for 10 minutes a day. We've already taken a brief look at the benefits and practices of meditation. And as it is its own kind of self-discipline and focus, it can only strengthen your self-discipline overall. The mutual benefit is that being more self-disciplined, you'll only get more out of your meditation.

- Here's another exercise to make you more self-disciplined. Make your bed. I know, some of you are balking in one direction or the other. Some people always do it, some people never do. For those who don't, consider the benefits. First, you've accomplished a small task, very first thing in the morning. That's good for self-efficacy. It puts you in a productive mindset. And as we've discussed, the environment mirrors the psyche. A messy bed makes for a messy mind, even if you're not there. Also, you never know who may come home with you, and you don't want to look like a slob.

- While you should have a healthy diet and lifestyle, don't neglect natural sugar intake. We know how too much or too little glucose can affect the brain. Glucose, you'll recall, carries energy to the brain and other organs, muscles, and bodily systems. When you're low on blood sugar, you risk losing motivation. But remember, everything in moderation!

Upon analysis, self-discipline seems rooted in three basic instincts: Self-preservation, self-assertion, and self-fulfillment.

1. Self-preservation takes focus off unimportant things and redirects it toward what is necessary, what is vital for survival. Those with this instinct tend not over overemphasize material goods and tend not to exploit others.
2. Those with a strong sense of self-assertion know what their value is but they're open to letting others speak as well. They're firm but gentle and resist abusive language or treatment of others.
3. Those who have or seek self-fulfillment are also resilient. Self-control urges this person on to facing challenges and

developing the skills necessary for success and happiness; in other words, self-fulfillment.

And these challenging but possibly necessary skills may include things like learning to dance or draw or any artistic pursuit which may take years to do well. These are the ultimate tests of self-discipline. Nobody's going to put that guitar in your hands and a gun to your head, after all ... you hope. That'd be pretty weird.

Self-control makes for a life of happy moderation, not living in the past or the future, neither wanting to much or failing to see when you've had enough.

DEVELOP THE SYSTEM TO BECOME A PRODUCTIVITY HERO!

There are a few modern systems that will help you get things done. We've leaned hard on the Pomodoro method, so let's take a look at a few more.

The *Getting Things Done* (GTD) starts with writing down anything and everything which needs to get done. We've done this before, but we'll rate them a bit differently. Classify them into six categories; current actions, current projects, areas of responsibility, 1-to-2-year goals. 3-to-5-year goals, and life goals.

Do the little ones first, get them out of the way and build up your self-efficacy and build up some momentum. As you might assume by now, break up the bigger projects into smaller milestones. Then proceed as we've done. It's the classifications which matter here. It's a good way to get control of short- and long-term goals. It's a little more advanced than doing a single project this way, but will put you in greater control of your life.

The *Zen to Done* (ZTD) approach is comparable to the Getting Things Done approach, but the Zen approach focuses on habits while the other focuses on the system. ZTD centers on the process, on the doing, in other words, while GTD focuses on creating a system and letting the system do the work.

GTD is a loosely structured timetable for task accomplishment. ZTD structures the day around three most important tasks and the week around major tasks. There's no five-year increment in the ZTD framework. ZTD uses simplification to focus you on essentials, more specific goals in tighter timelines.

ZTD's focus on our habits is central, and there are habits every ZTD master seems to evince. They capture ideas, notes, and tasks so they're not forgotten. They make quick decisions and don't procrastinate. They set most important tasks for each day. They do one task at a time without distractions, no multi-tasking. They keep simple lists and check them daily. They have organized environments with a place for everything. They review their goals and systems regularly and reduce them to which are essential. They set and keep routines and they work passionately at work for which they are passionate.

Sound familiar? Everything we've been working on leads us to this, prepares us for it, makes it not only possible but almost simplistic!

The system known as *Don't Break the Chain* was apparently inspired by comedian Jerry Seinfeld. Not surprisingly, it focuses on creative success. The story goes that the comic bought a calendar and drew a thick red X through every day in which he wrote new material. The idea was that if he didn't write any new material on a given day, he would break the chain of X marks. It may sound simplistic, but it uses almost all the techniques we've discussed in one easy-to-use system. It's a time-log, it's accountability, it's visualizing, it's motivational. X out every day that you do something to accomplish your goal and don't break the chain.

And what is it with airline food, am I right?

You can modify the system though. If you're on vacation, use blue instead of red. Vacationing is part of refreshing your productive cycle, after all. And an X is still an X. But keep it red as much as you can! You can also allow yourself a few gaps in a month, but not two in a row, and not more than one per week. Then hang that calendar in a prominent place, where you can see it, be reminded by it, be inspired by it.

This method won't be great for complex time management or Pomodoro-style milestone projects, just a continued advance toward a single thing. This one is great for self-discipline, because you do that in so many different ways every day, and they're all steps on a single journey. You might also keep several calendars, one for self-discipline, one for personal projects, one for professional projects. You can use the same color-coding system for each to keep them easy to follow.

The *Daily Trifecta* method focuses on three things per day so that those tasks are all completed by the end of the day. It's a good method for short-term goals and for any Pomodoro-style construct.

The *MOSCOW* method breaks up tasks into four categories of differing value: Must-have (M), should have (S), could have (C), and would have (W). Ranking your tasks this way will help you prioritize them, organize them, and then get them done!

Whichever one you choose, the method of choice should be friction-free, adaptable to your personal needs, be easy to learn, encourage working with others, and compatible with other systems. All of the above fit the bill perfectly. Try one, or try a few of them. Combine them as they might serve you best.

Now let's take a closer look at applying these systems to any and every aspect of your life!

IV

REACHING YOUR
UNLIMITED POTENTIAL

HANDLING THE DIFFERENT AREAS OF YOUR LIFE

DROP THE FIXED MINDSET AND START DEVELOPING A GROWTH MINDSET

There's no single way to reach your unlimited potential, of course. There's no magic key. But, like any big task, you can use the set of skills you've already been developing to achieve this daunting task. And it'll be an ongoing task. As it is with self-discipline, it's a constant forge, and you'll either be constantly improving it or risking it backsliding and yourself along with it.

Let's start this section, about reaching your unlimited potential by breaking the big task down to smaller tasks. It works every time.

Perhaps the first milestone for this project will be to look at where potential lies, and that's in the mind. Your thoughts are central to the direction your life will take; we've seen that in a number of ways. Lack of self-efficacy, negative self-talk, and a variety of other unhealthy mental habits stem from your brain, which we've already taken a look at. But what about the actual thoughts? We've looked at the different types of memory, the different ways emotion affects thought. Now let's dig deeper into that influence, and how you can put it all together and start applying it for even more concrete results (if you've been applying these practices and exercises, my guess is that you've already seen a few, even small ones).

So, onward to thoughts. Thoughts can be constructive or destructive to your self-improvement, as we've seen. But thoughts don't exist in a vacuum, they're generated by a mindset. To understand your thoughts and their effects on your behavior and your life, you have to go deeper still, into the complexities of the mindset.

There are basically two mindsets; a *growth* or a *fixed* mindset. Their nature is intuitive. A growth mindset believes a set of skills or even a situation can be changed, improved, that a thing can *grow*. A fixed mindset generally sees things as static, unchangeable, inevitable, that a thing is *fixed*.

Not surprisingly, those with a fixed mindset tend to be depressed and tend toward failure. Those with a growth mindset tend toward satisfaction and success. The good news is that you (or anyone) can change their mindset and thereby change your thought process, going on to change your life.

Qualities like willpower, courage, creativity, diligence, and good communication skills are learned, not innate, as we've seen. Those with a growth mindset are better prepared and more likely to embrace this and to excel at those qualities.

Those with a fixed mindset tend to avoid challenges, give up easily, perceive effort as worthless or a waste of time. They tend to ignore feedback and are threatened by the success of others.

In contrast, those with a growth mindset embrace challenges, they even look forward to them. They persist when challenged, they don't give up easily. They tend to see effort as the path to mastery. They learn from criticism and believe lessons are inspirational and will lead to success.

In one study of 128 children 10 to 11 years of age, two groups were given identical math problems to solve. One group was encouraged with, "You're doing very well. You must be smart!" In the other group, they encouraged with, "You're doing well. You must be trying hard!" The test went on a few more steps, and the final results were clear. The children encouraged for their innate intelligence fared less well than those praised for the growth mindset of trying hard.

Researchers believe this is so because those who's believe in their own intelligence didn't feel they had to try as hard, and so they did less well. Those praised for their attempts responded to that praise by trying even harder, and thus they did better.

You might recognize the connection to the mindsets of optimism and pessimism. And those mindsets are also not innate and can be changed with self-discipline and knowledge. This is important as it relates to our failures; whether we think we can learn from them or merely be defeated by them, for example.

People with a growth mindset tend to bounce back from failure, as we've seen, and they generally come back stronger. They learn from their failures. In fact, the old saying goes something like, *"You learn more from your failures than your successes."* That is a growth mindset in a nutshell. People with fixed mindsets seem to believe that nothing can be learned from success at all. Growth minded people believe that failure leads to success, but those with a fixed mindset tend to see one failure as proof of a pattern of failure, one which cannot be reversed.

Changing this one link in the chain can be invaluable, even crucial, to your personal growth. At the moment of failure, deliberately choose to adopt a growth mindset, even if you never had one before. Force yourself to be an optimist, no matter how difficult or futile that may seem. It's well within anybody's ability to control their mindset, their thoughts, their behaviors, their goals, their achievements, their lives. They just have to see it that way. Hopefully, *you* do.

But these mindsets are related to still one more phenomenon; the self-fulfilling prophecy.

Famed automaker and American titan Henry Ford once said, "Whether you think you can, or you think you can't ... you're right." Research bears this out. People tend to fall victim to the limits they impose upon themselves. If a person believes themselves to be a perpetual loser, they are not likely to have many successes. They will self-sabotage their efforts in the variety of ways we've already looked at. The belief becomes reality, and a self-fulfilling prophecy is fulfilled.

But I'll bet you've already figured that the reverse is also true. The growth-minded person tells themselves that failure can be surmounted, that they are successes at their core. These people are more willing to take chances and reap the benefits of accomplishing new and challenging tasks.

So, know what your general mindset is. Make a few lists, rank the things in your life which you have accomplished, gave up on accomplishing, or still hope to accomplish. Which list is longer, which is shorter? If you have a long list of things you gave up but a short list of things you have to accomplish, you'll know that reflects a fixed mindset, and that's been limiting you.

Once you change your mindset for the better, your whole life will change for the better!

And, like the other mindsets, be diligent! A person can change their mindset deliberately, from fixed to growth, but it can also work the other way. A person with a growth mindset may be dissuaded through years of failure and fall into a fixed mindset if they're not diligent, maintaining self-discipline. Support partners can be essential tools in this case (as in so many of the things we've discussed in this book).

New neuroscientific advances now show that the brain is more flexible than previously thought. Neurons can change over time under the influence of experience. New connections can grow, and old connections can be strengthened. The insulation which speeds up transmission of impulses can be restored or built up! Furthermore, we can influence this growth with concrete actions, things anybody can do, and a lot of them are right in this book: Better nutrition and sleep habits, employing sound strategies, asking the right questions and setting the right goals, practicing heathy habits like reading or playing a musical instrument.

As you can see, changing your mindset to a growth-oriented perspective can actually improve your brain function, and that in turn will help everything else you think and do. This positive cycle feeds itself and an upward spiral is accelerated.

DON'T DISMISS YOUR FEELINGS, YOUR TOPMOST PRIORITY IS YOURSELF

Making yourself a top priority means employing a variety of the techniques you've already used. But it's important to be deliberate about applying them to every facet of your daily life. And since we're harder on ourselves than on others the area of self-care is of vital importance. Add to that the incredible stress in our daily lives, the processed food, the economic demands, the overwhelming amounts of information that pour into our brains, self-care is both the first thing people forget and the last thing they can afford to forgo.

Healthy sleep habits, better diet, daily exercise, self-discipline, the Pomodoro technique, all are great ways to self-care. Abandon perfectionism, practice self-sympathy. Avoid negative self-talk and overthinking. Learn a new skill.

Self-care for students is also especially important. Their schedules are often packed with scholastic, extra-scholastic, and lots of recreational activity. They work hard and they play hard, draining their resources at every turn. Additionally, students seem more prone to procrastination and overthinking than other groups taken as a whole.

But experts recommend other tips and tricks specifically for self-care.

Just say *no*. We've touched on it briefly before, but bears repeating here. Our lives are so filled with people who need us for one thing or another, we're pressured to over-perform. And it's true that a positive mindset is apt to take advantage of opportunities which come along, it's important to be selective, have discretion. You won't have enough time or resources to do everything you're asked to do in life. That will reduce your ability to do things you're already committed to. We've looked at making lists and prioritizing, and you should employ that technique here. Remember that tasks may be urgent or important, both urgent and important, urgent but not important, important but not urgent, and neither urgent nor important. So, dedicate yourself to the things which are important and urgent first. Because of its effects on your long-term goals and because of its effect on your immediate performance, self-care is both important and urgent.

We haven't talked much about taking vacations, though they are excellent rewards to encourage the completion of a big task. Here, it's an even more vital concept. Self-care trips are really powerful ways to maintain your physical and mental wellbeing. Think about spending the weekend at a hot springs resort or a spa, where you can dedicate yourself entirely to self-care, body, and mind. Camping, golf trips, meditation retreats, there is all manner of self-care destinations you might consider. You may also think about a trip to see family (though that might not reduce your stress at all).

Emotional support pets are very popular, and for good reason. They have a calming, soothing influence. They're a little bit of nature right there in the house with you. They can be sounding boards and sources of support. They're loving. Taking care of a pet is in itself a huge task which you break down into smaller tasks of upkeep and interaction. Just the act of having and maintaining a pet will help you defeat procrastination and overthinking, in fact. Go back and take a look, reread a few things with pet ownership in mind, you'll see what I mean.

It really doesn't matter what kind of animal it is. Whatever appeals to you. Some people just love to stroke the fur of a dog or cat or bunny rabbit. Others find solace in the colors and languid motion of exotic fish; others adore their pet birds. Teaching a parrot to talk is a classic example of the Pomodoro technique and will in itself serve just about every practice we've analyzed.

Being organized is especially important to self-care, because being disorganized is the source of such constant stress and confusion in our daily lives. Self-care is hardly doable without being reasonably well-organized.

Cooking at home is an amazing self-care technique. Not only will the food be as pure and natural as you make it, and it will taste better, but you have the benefit of doing the cooking. Cooking incorporates so much of what we've looked at, combining virtually every technique. When you cook, you're learning a new skill, that's good for the brain. Your self-efficacy and positive thought process are escalated. Small tasks are rewarded with deliciousness, plus the pride of accomplishments. It reduces perfectionism but motivates organization and effort and self-sympathy. It's healthier, and it can have a meditative effect. It's a lot more economical too, which not only reduces the related stress but gives you a sense of control over the economy.

Remember to schedule time for self-care every day. Don't break the chain on this one, it's too important.

Self-care is crucially important to those in recovery from or managing a serious illness. Be it recovery from an accident or dealing with a sudden or chronic illness, self-care is at the heart of any recovery regiment. And there are specific things you might think about if you're employing self-care for this purpose.

Interestingly, facing a medical crisis is very much the kind of big tasks we've been looking at throughout this book, the kind of task you've been training for. It employs almost all the things we've discussed, from a growth mindset to the Pomodoro technique. Recovering from a broken leg requires successfully completing a series of milestones; learning to use crutches, getting out of the cast, physical therapy. Recovery from cancer means surgery or radiation, perhaps rounds of chemotherapy; each of them are a milestone to be completed toward the ultimate goal of recovery. There are lots of other now-familiar techniques which are employed (better sleep and diet, more exercise, meditation, self-sympathy, positive thinking, visualizing).

But let's take a closer look at a few concrete ways to self-care if you're facing a significant recovery process.

First off, you'll definitely want to focus on your strengths and on solving problems. Abandon the past and focus on the future. It's true that we've emphasized living in the present and abandoning the past or the future as a way to beat overthinking. But remember too that the future is a great motivator, and it's key to assembling our long-term plans. In this case, lean on the future to get you through the present.

You'll also want to stay focused on your life. Take the focus away from your disease. This won't be easy. You'll need all your self-discipline to resist being obsessed with it; a life-threatening disease, sure, but even a broken leg can dominate every second of your waking thought. It itches under the cast, your football days are over, it may hurt every time it rains or be a constant pain your whole life. There's a lot to worry about.

But draw on the skills you learned in mediation. And remember habits, and how it's better to replace one with its opposite. Replace your focus on the disease or injury with your focus on a loved one, visualize a dream of future success or happiness. Focus on that one thing, at first for five minutes a day, then ten, and so on. Remove distraction and clutter. Anyone can do it.

People facing recovery should pay particular attention to hygiene. Slipping hygiene can be a sign of helplessness, depression, giving up. See friends too, as increasing isolation indicate the same things.

Do one thing you enjoy every day, something for pure pleasure. Watch an episode of your favorite TV show, take a hot bath.

One thing which is often overlooked in the realm of self-care, be it from injury or illness or just of the basic, general variety of self-care.

Clothes.

Clothes are ubiquitous in our society. They signal our status, our priorities, they express who we are. They are like an environment which we carry around everywhere we go. It mirrors our psyche.

If self-care is your aim (or whatever your aim, really) you should take a look at what you're wearing and what you *should* be wearing.

Clothes can either serve to make you more confident (on the job or on a date) or more relaxed (at home after work, on vacation). Dress for the occasion! It's a lot easier to be comfortable in a bathrobe at home, but a lot more difficult to be confident in one at the office.

Clothes reflect who you are and can affect the way you feel about yourself. They can also affect the way others feel about you. Clothing is a vital connection to others and to the world at large.

Clothes are also a good motivator to socialize a bit more. Imagine being all dressed up with nowhere to go.

Also, changing from work clothes to your personal clothes helps you maintain boundaries. You want to prevent your work life from dominating your personal life. Time off is a big part of self-care, after all.

Work shorter hours if you can. In this competitive society, the 8-hour workday is increasingly rare. But to work much more than that causes lack of focus, burnout, a less-impressive result, and that contributes to a downward spiral. But this can happen without us even knowing it. Outside of a workplace setting, in the new gig economy, it's easier and even more necessary to work longer hours. And in the office, workers often stay late or come in early or even forego lunch to get things done. But as we've seen, these overachievers can easily become underachievers, in this case from sheer burnout. Too many hours at the desk leads to all kinds of physical maladies, from knee and back problems to eye strain and circulatory issues, it's physically dangerous. Work shorter hours if you can and get up and walk around a bit every hour or so to prevent blood clots.

To this end, a lot of people now work at stand-up desks. There are a variety of models, all of them easily adjustable for sitting or standing. It's apparently great for posture, overall comfort, productivity and stamina. Hey, Ernest Hemingway wrote standing up, and we all remember him.

But to get back to working shorter hours, standing up or not, consider scheduling fewer hours to get the job done, that will motivate you to spend less time working. A lot of people believe 35 hours should be the max. I personally work about 70 hours a week.

To make the most out of fewer work hours, let's take a look at a few time-tested rules for corporate time management as it relates to holding meetings.

TIME MANAGEMENT FOR THE CORPORATE WORLD

A way to deal with your own struggles with a busy schedule is to have *theme* days. By that, I mean each day might be set aside for a certain type of activity. You might focus on organization on Mondays, scheduling on Tuesdays, personal interaction on Wednesdays, phone calls on Thursdays, organizing the next week's plans on Friday.

But meetings are by far one of the hardest things to manage in the corporate world. There are different personalities with different tasks and different abilities. Meetings tend to go long and that derails careful time planning. Estimates are that workers spend about 15% of their workweek in meetings. Here are some brilliant ways to keep your meetings running smoothly, efficiently, and quickly.

Keep your meetings to five–minutes. The so-called *five-minute rule* illustrates that most people can get their point across in about half a minute. Six people can report their progress and digest their next moves in that time. If five minutes is too few, make it the minimum and ten minutes the max, maybe fifteen. Nothing more than that. The five-minute rule is golden to the efficient corporate manager.

No meeting should go longer than an hour. No meeting has that many people making that many points.

Set one day aside as a *no meetings* day. Wednesday is good, as every-body should be embroiled in the tasks they were set on Monday. They'll be reporting on Thursday and Friday anyway, so why not give them and yourself a break and let you all knuckle down and get the work done? This will also break up the drudgery of the workweek.

End early if you can. Schedule an hour but shoot to wind up at the 50-minute mark. It sets an example for the others to beat their deadlines too. And it gives them an extra ten minutes to get out of meeting mode and back into work mode. It gives you ten extra minutes too, for some quick meditation or to allow for unexpected complexities which may come up.

Don't start your meetings on the hour. It sounds counterintuitive, but it's true. Standard meeting times lull employees into a state of complacency and they can easily wind up coming in late. Making your meeting at 8:19 am sharp will make the meeting seem more important and less routine. It will challenge your employees to be detail oriented, and to show up on time. And if it's a midday meeting, some of your employees may legitimately be running late due to ongoing business. The off-hour meeting time allows them a margin without actually being late.

The *three-bounce rule* is known to most good managers. It states that as soon as a single topic has had three exchanges back-and-forth, the subject is tabled for another meeting. This prevents the subject from dominating the meeting and derailing the other important subjects. It's the cousin to the five-minute rule.

Don't neglect impact; the impact of one person's work has on the team, for good or ill. Every action has an equal and opposite reaction, after all. Actions have consequences, make sure your team members know that.

Always have an agenda. This will keep your meetings running smoothly and on time and prevent anything from getting lost or forgotten. An agenda will tell you how much time you have to spend on each subject. Time it out, in fact. You've got an hour for the meeting and five subjects? None get more than twenty-minutes. Make sure that allows time for unexpected interruptions.

Speaking of interruptions, smartphones are a big distraction throughout the day, so consider making a rule that smartphones are not allowed in meetings.

Employees generally maintain either a *makers* schedule or a *managers* schedule. Managers are used to taking meetings, but makers are used to working more and meeting less, if at all. For a maker, a midday schedule can punch a hole in their productive day, seriously interrupting the workflow and reducing productivity. Managers do little but take meetings. So, if you're scheduling a meeting with a maker, do it first thing in the morning so they can get back to their logo design or writing project. Your managers should be at your disposal just about any time.

All this being said, some meetings should be longer. Your staff will appreciate the perfunctory, efficient meetings, yes. But they also long to reconnect on a certain human level, and the big meetings allow for that. Give them a chance to gossip a little, catch up how the other's wives or husbands or children are doing. Let them be personal in the work context. But do this only when it seems reasonable, not with every little meeting. And when you do let them indulge (and indulge yourself too) keep it from going too long. Ten minutes or so should do it. Then, it's back to work!

Speaking of distractions like Smartphones, there are other common external office distractions you're going to have to keep an eye on, as much as you can. Internal distractions include fatigue, illness, personal problems or concerns, and daydreaming. There's little you can do here but gently support your team member and encourage them to get whatever professional help they need. That's good for them and it's good for your business.

Distractions in the workplace make for between 70% to an astonishing 99% of office employees report feeling distracted. The average employee is distracted roughly 56 times a day. The same studies also tell us that the average worker takes roughly 2 hours over the course of the day transitioning between distractions and actual work.

Distractions take their toll on the workers too. Of those surveyed, 54% of corporate makers or managers report that they feel that they're not performing as well as they should while 50% report being significantly less productive. A full 20% report being unable to reach their full career potential. Greater distractions have been shown to have a negative effect on memory, too.

Mobile phone use, the internet, and gossip are the three leading causes, though not the only ones. Of course, people go on their mobile phones largely to use the internet, so that particular distraction is particularly troublesome.

The internet is a huge distraction, but it's a big part of the workday for so many managers and makers, it's impossible to ban them; ditto, smartphones. But there are apps you can install in your office computers, such as *Strict Workflow* and *StayFocusd*, can limit your workers' access to certain, more distracting websites.

Another common distraction is chatty coworkers. Certainly, you want them to be friendly and to interact freely, but the focus inevitably turns to personal subjects and gossip. This can lead to rumors, feuds, toxic feelings which can become contagious and spread throughout your team. It's best to limit this if you can. But don't be overly authoritarian either. Correct them if you need to, and then be firm and reasonable. Explain that you'd like to get the most out of their efforts during work hours, and other things can be discussed outside work hours, if they must be. And always discourage rumors and gossip. That is never acceptable behavior, especially not in an office setting. It's tempting, and it's fun, but remind them of the benefits of self-discipline and the drawbacks of negativity. Even if they don't agree, my guess is that they'd take the hint.

Avoid office politics too. Make it clear to all that you run a meritocracy. Praise and reward go to those who perform based on results, not based on the person. Sounds familiar, right? Good.

An offshoot of this is the background noise generated by workers who are too loud. Whether they're on the phone with a client or chatting with a coworker, the sheer volume of these voices can become a distraction. It's a more common complaint than you might think among corporate workers today. Try to keep a library rule in the office and limit any chat to a low volume, a short time limit, and a high-value priority. If it's important, make it quick and keep it quiet. Loud eating is a similar annoyance.

Limit personal visits to the office; spouses with children or even pets are very disruptive to the office workflow. You can still have office birthday parties and corporate picnics where everybody is welcome. But office time is for office business.

It's a lot to look after, but I think you'll find it's worthwhile. Studies show that 75% of workers report getting more done with fewer distractions, and 57% of people report feeling motivated to do their very best. Fifty-one percent reported feeling more confident, and 44%

believe their work is improved. Those are impressive numbers but think of all that productivity you're losing if you're not managing your office distractions efficiently.

More practical tips for dealing with distractions include noise-cancelling headphones, which also combats another big distraction; loud coworkers.

We've talked about distractions at work and how to deal with them, but more and more of us work from home, and that's not likely to change. So how do we deal with the distractions of home while doing the work of the office?

Family will have constant demands on you, and of all the people it's hardest to say *no* to, it's your beloved spouse and adorable rug-rats. But you're going to have to be firm, set them all down, and explain that you've got a workday, 8 am to 5 pm or whatever it is. During that time, you are not to be disturbed. Maybe now you're seeing how important it is to train yourself to be able to say *no*, because this will be the greatest test. And it won't just happen once, you may have to remind them from time to time … throughout the day.

Same goes for your neighbors. Your jolly neighbor may spot you at home and assume you've got time for a chat. Kindly correct him. Hey, if you could say no to your family, you can probably disappoint Stanley and Ida next store or across the street.

You might consider inviting your neighbors to enjoy a barbeque to make up for how much time you spent working. That'll have all the benefits of cooking, socializing, and recreating.

Housework is another distraction that's more particular to the home. Offices are generally cleaned by a crew in the middle of the night. But avoid housework as a distraction. Hopefully you have a support partner in your family who can fill the breach. Even your kids may be willing to chip in and help. That would be a good lesson for them in almost everything we've looked at in this book, from self-discipline to self-efficacy to a sense of connection between themselves and their environment.

Food and drink are other home-oriented distractions. You may have a snack machine or a soda machine in the break room, but you probably don't have a fridge full of yummy leftovers, a variety of beverages, hot tea filling the air. Your senses are hard to beat, and they will motivate you to be distracted. Don't be. Hey, nothing worthwhile is ever easy, right? If you backslide here, you'll get less done and put on extra weight, itself the source of all kinds of bad behaviors. Don't say you weren't warned!

MAKING MONEY IS SOMETHING THAT YOU SHOULD ENJOY DOING

Let's be honest. Business is about profit. That profit should not come from the suffering of others, sacrifices and rewards should be evenly distributed. But in the end, business makes money, or they fail. And good corporate management means ensuring the company's success, not its failure. The corporate success is your big long-term task, everything else you do professionally is a milestone. Some of those are so big they're their own big tasks, which are broken down, and so forth.

But money carries baggage for a lot of people. They may have feelings of guilt over having too much or shame over having too little. It changes some and can ruin others. Yet it's something we absolutely need. And it's part of the cycle of positive behavior. Money means success, freedom to enjoy the finer things in life. It allows us to help those in want or need. It allows us to extricate ourselves from emergencies, bringing stability and a lack of stress. As much as we hate to admit it, it's what a lot of us are working so hard for.

There are basically two direction money flows, in and out. It may come in as income, dividends or investment profits, inheritance, fluke things like lottery wins. It goes out in the form of expenses like food and shelter, transportation and necessities, luxuries and amusement, taxes and loan penalties.

Investments and savings represent a strange dichotomy. The cash may move out of your bank account, but it moves into your stock portfolio, so it isn't really spent. But it's still not in your bank account either. Savings, on the other hand, represents money that moves in and doesn't move out. Savings are harder to come by these days, and it's a crucial part of financial stability. Most Americans asked today report having less than $400 dollars in the bank.

If you're finances are slipping out of your control, always fall back on what you've learned here. If paying off a credit card is a big task, break it up Pomodoro style, and tackle it in smaller chunks (as long as they meet the minimum monthly payment, of course).

The first thing to do to tackle your personal finances, you may not be surprised to hear, is to make a series of lists, logs, and plans. The first thing you need is a budget. Write down how much you earn in a month and add it up, then how much you spend; on necessities like rent and food, and on luxuries. If your luxury column is too high, simply reduce spending on those things. Sacrifice them until your finances are back on track. Then you can return to one or two of them, if you still want to.

Common luxuries you can surely cut off the list (temporarily) is eating out. Homemade food tastes better than prepared food, and you get all the benefits of cooking; the meditative and creative and organizational skills, the instant gratification, the boom in self-confidence.

Allocate about 20% of your income to financial priorities, and 30% toward lifestyle spending. But stick to that and don't let the thirty become thirty-five, forty, or even more. Since your rent or mortgage is probably about 30% of your income, your personal spending should be necessarily limited.

Cut those credit card bills by paying a certain amount over the minimum every month. Otherwise you'll never get out from under them. While you're at it, cut cable. You're paying a lot for things you don't watch. Why not skip and watch just what you want on YouTube? At least you can skip the ad in 5 ... 4 ... 3 ... 2 ...

You may want to put the cards away for a while. Don't make a bad situation worse. Commit to going to a cash-only basis for one week a month. Stay away from those credit cards!

Plan to put something away for savings every month. Make it the same amount every month and make you deposit on the same day every month. You can create a special savings account and then transfer the money online, so a visit to the bank isn't even necessary.

Some people enjoy a spending fast, where they set about to spend nothing for a given period. Can you go two days? Three? Five? Even if you can't do more than two, you're still saving.

Don't commit to any recurring monthly charges. You can lose track and wind up spending monthly on things you don't need or perhaps even want. If you have ongoing charges, make a list of them and track them by expense and value. Think about reducing your current ongoing charges by half or more if you can. The savings will add up automatically if you just cut loose that Netflix subscription.

Another good way to watch your finances is good ol'-fashioned bargain hunting. They're around more and more. Smartphone apps are dedicated to saving you money on car insurance, nights out, all manner of items you may be spending too much for. There are also retail outlet stores which offer heavily discounted merchandise. When grocery shopping, always keep an eye out for the sale deals. And take your local supermarket on a savings club card if they have one. You could save up to or more than 20% per visit to the grocery store.

Like a lot of the things we've discussed, being good with money takes practice, but there are lots of good ways to do it. And the results are sure to make your life and your other efforts a lot easier and more stress-free.

Managing money, as much as anything we've discussed, requires a support friend. This person could be your spouse, your business manager, your accountant, a friend, or a family member. But you'll need help somewhere along the line, for sure. This particular long-term task may require more than one friend, but a whole support network. Your spouse and children, if you have them, should be involved in the campaign, helping to save too.

Here are yet a few more handy tricks when it comes to money:

Never cosign a loan. It will corrode a family relationship, and it could destroy your credit and cost you a fortune. This time it should be easy to say *no*. That being said, a lot of parents cosign loans for their newly adult children; first cars, apartment leases. But this is not the usual and even than can be fraught with difficulties.

If you're a student, go after every federal loan or grant or scholarship you can find. Avoid student loans like the plague if you can. If you're already struggling with payments like these, look into federal plans for assistance or other repayment options.

LIVING A LEISURE LIFE ON TOP OF YOUR RESPONSIBILITIES

And all this planning could and should lead you to a bit more free time. But how you spend that free time is important to your overall plan. If you live healthily on the weekdays and then go out and trash yourself on the weekends, you will suffer a reduction of productivity later.

Research indicates that adults in the US enjoy roughly 40 hours of time away from work. Men and women seem to spend about five hours a day in so-called *free time*. This is time outside of the responsibilities of household chores, work, curricular and religious activities. Watching TV, sitting in the hot tub, whatever.

Free time tends to draw us to activities or events, but not all are of equal value. When presented with a free time opportunity, ask yourself, "Will this give me a good story to tell? Will it change me in some positive way? Will it allow me to relax and support my personal relationships? Is it challenging? Does it fill me with a sense of wonder, fill my heart with the milk of human kindness? Does it improve my social standing? Will it bring comfort or happiness to someone I love?"

If the answer is *yes*, you should definitely go. If not, give them stronger consideration and more discretion.

NO MAN IS AN ISLAND, THE RELATIONSHIPS YOU BUILD ARE NECESSARY FOR YOUR LIFE

One of the best ways to strengthen any relationship, is to be a good listener. It's been said that the best conversationalist you'll ever meet only talks about one subject ... you. And this is largely true. First of all, we're a self-centered culture, and very few people do anything but go on and on about themselves anyway. Instead of competing for their attention, which may not be worth having in the first place, just give them what they want. Ask them about themselves, deflect questions about yourself, and be a good listener. It doesn't do much good if you're constantly asking question after question, interrupting the answers you're supposed to be listening to. Just listen.

Still, that's not as easy as it sounds. Our competitive environment encourages us to speak up for ourselves, to toot our own horns, to think the most of ourselves, to make the most of ourselves and every opportunity. But a lot of that means presenting yourself as a caring, interested person, somebody not bent on making the most of every opportunity but allowing the other person to do the same.

It does take surprising will and self-control. And like all the things we've talked about so far, it requires a certain depth of understanding. And there's more to the art of listening than you may know.

First, there will always be some discrepancy between what a person intends to say and how you interpret that. It's a natural drawback of language. And it's made worse by emails and text, which lack all the subtleties and reactive possibilities of a live conversation where you can at least hear the person's voice and see their face. There's no better way to be misunderstood than to send an email or text.

Language is important because it is what best represents us. You can't judge a book by its cover, they say, but a person's language is what is printed on the pages of their soul.

And there are two varieties of the art of listening. There is passive and active listening, and you must know which is best and which you lean toward in order to make the most of your relationship.

The passive listener doesn't really listen, they just tolerate their time to wait until they can deliver their position. They're not about to be swayed or really even engaged. The active listener takes into account what the other is saying, digesting it, ready to be moved by it.

It's impossible to miss the parallel between a growth mindset or a fixed mindset. The passive listener is likely to have a fixed mindset, unwilling to consider the possibilities of change. The active listener, change-oriented, is vastly more likely to be of a growth mindset.

Spending time with friends and family is crucial to strengthen your relationships, for obvious reasons. These are the strongest relationships you have. Your most formative influences were first your family and then your friends, so these are the groups who are best served to be your support network, the cradle of your non-professional life.

Such an intimate support network, as opposed to a work support network of friendly coworkers, offers a sense of belonging, security, increased self-worth. It is said to reduce your stress levels (if you're not in my family!) and all jokes aside, studies bear this out.

Romantic relationships, like familial relationships and longtime friendships, will have highs and lows over the years as the individuals experience their own changes. So, you really should be as willing to be tolerant of the other person's changes, as you would expect that person would do for you, Remember the so-called *Golden Rule: Do unto others as you would have them to unto you.*

Relationships are unique, so each has to be dealt with on its own terms. If you're willing to deal with the other person in your life on their terms, you've got a good chance. If you're only willing to deal on your own terms, you might wind up alone. But your partner will face the same challenges, so think of it as facing them together.

Relationships of all sorts are about two things; feelings and communications. So often, we feel one thing but say another, to protect ourselves or because we lack the skills to say what we truly feel. That's not as easy as it sounds either. For example, you may have respect for a person, but that's not enough if you act out and treat them disrespectfully. You have to show respect, or your feelings are irrelevant to that person. It's not enough to love, you have to show love, communicate it successfully.

The flipside of that coin isn't showing it but receiving that feeling. A person may simply not feel loved or understood. You always have to keep in mind, not only what you are feeling and perhaps failing to communicate, but what the other is hearing and perhaps failing to process.

If you disagree, remain respectful. Don't personalize it. Think of the emphasis on the results of the task or on the value of the worker. The healthier focus is on the thing, not the person. And this only makes sense because a thing cannot be insecure or insulted or lash out, but a person will be more than ready to do so. So be resolved to be as respectful as you can in disagreements. Don't insist on being right but do express yourself so you can avoid overthinking later!

For a successful relationship, don't cut yourself off from other interests and relationships. A happy life is a well-rounded life. The more which enriches you outside the relationship, the more you can bring to the relationship.

And beware of any relationship partner who tries to separate you from your family or your friends, unless they truly are abusive in a criminal sense. The concept of a *splitter*, or a *wedge personality*, is a well-known element in relationships. This is a personality who seeks to isolate and control the other person, destroying their trust in their previous relationships.

Remember that there's a difference between *falling* in love and *staying* in love. The first may be chaotic and random, but the second is almost always the result of a determined effort from both parties.

Otherwise, everything in this book covers romance as if it were a big, long-term goal (a life's love) made up of a series of goals and milestones (dating, engagement, marriage, staying married) which are rewarded and require planning and a positive mindset and so on. Tilt it just the right way, you've just read the best dating manual ever! To touch on just a few, the techniques we've learned which come into play most in the romantic arena include scheduled commitment (weekends, celebrations), learning new skills (which you share, like dance classes or wine tasting), recreation and self-care (and mutual care, in this case), volunteer together (at a food bank or helping with a city cleaning initiative),

Do things together that benefit others. Communicate clearly and respectfully but also take note of the physical cues you may get from the other. And be honest, as your body language is likely to give you away and you don't want to be rightfully called out as a liar.

Beware of stress, which may make you misread what your partner is saying or conveying. In times of stress, it might be best to avoid going too deep. Wait until you're both calmer and more reasonable. Remember the influence of emotion on our behavior and act accordingly.

As with the other things we've looked at, it's crucial to abandon perfectionism in a relationship. Nobody's perfect, and no coupling is absolutely perfect.

A HEARTY SPIRITUAL LIFE

Well, maybe God is perfect, which is one of the most attractive aspects of religion. It not only provides regiment to our lives, and socialization, education, even philosophy. Some focus more on the ethereal aspect, others on the more earthbound social aspect. Either way, it can be very good for developing personal skills and becoming a better, happier, and more well-rounded person.

The benefits of spirituality include reassurance, a clearer view of perfectionism and its faults but at the same time fostering a stronger sense of self-efficacy and value and that encourages positive self-talk. Spirituality can provide meaning, something to focus on in the way of meditation. It helps foster sympathy for others and connections to others, and generates a growth mindset.

Research shows that religious people recovered faster from various types of heart surgery than those of weaker faith or no faith at all! Those who attend religious services seem to live longer than those who don't.

To seek a more spiritually grounded life, any of the major organized religions will give you ample opportunities. There's no time to survey them here, but your libraries, bookstores, and internet outlets are filled with books on all of them, and from every different angle.

Once you find the religion which best expresses your beliefs, participate. Jesus said, "Faith without works is dead." So, get out there and act on that faith. You'll find it has every benefit of the many tips and techniques we've already discussed, and for the same reasons. It's great for positive self-talk, socialization, gratification, focus, stress reduction, and more!

Make sure the organization you join is more spiritual than an organization, if you take my meaning. A church may ask for up to 10% of your income as a tithing, or contribution to the functioning of the church, and most small churches need that. A legitimate organization will encourage you to get closer to your family and friends. Any organization that asks for more than 10% or tries to separate you from your family and friends is to be avoided at all costs.

Become comfortable with the notion of prayer. It's not so different than having a support partner, only that might be the like of Christ Jesus Himself! You've got a sounding board and a mentor.

Reading religious texts has all the benefits of reading anything else. It stimulates the brain, it invigorates the creative spirit, it encourages focus in the face of infinite distraction.

Share your experiences and views with others. Give voice to it and make it real. This is especially potent in the context of the Abrahamic religions, Judaism especially.

Well, we started deep inside ourselves, and we wound up in the heavens themselves. Hopefully, you've learned a lot along the way. If something seems less clear, don't worry. There was a lot to digest. Go back and read it again, just the relevant sections if you like. This book was written for you, so by all means make the most of it!

CONCLUSION

Congratulations! You've just been exposed to the latest and best information about procrastination and overthinking and a good deal more than that. You've got a handful of tips and trick to apply this knowledge to your everyday life. You're now able to adapt a different mindset, a better perspective, with greater understanding of the challenges you and others face in your daily personal and professional lives. You've got everything you need to live a happier, more successful, and more fulfilling life. You've got the tools to correct a downward spiral, to reverse negative self-talk and a fixed mindset. You're ready try meditation, you can see the benefits of a healthier lifestyle. And everything you now know can be applied to your life immediately. Other than a few little materials, you've got everything you need to correct a lifetime of negativity and create the life you've always wanted. One of Albert Einstein's guiding principles was that if you can visualize it, it is possible. Think about that, and start seeing what your future is going to be like once you apply the data, lessons, and techniques you learned in this book.

We started by digging into the deepest center of your core thoughts and beliefs. Then worked outward to virtually every part of your body. We went further, through your clothes and your immediate environment to the people around you, personal, and professional. We looked at the mutual influence we all share, then reached further out to social ramification, to a worldwide pandemic of procrastination and overthinking, the negative self-talk, and limiting mindset which are true for people all over the world. We went to the Far East for remedies like meditation. We transcended Earth and looked to the heavens for support, to India for the wisdom of Buddhism.

And it all comes back to you; your life on every level. You've got what it takes to improve your life and to help others improve their lives. I'd wish you good luck, but you no longer need it. You've already got everything you need to take the next steps toward a brighter future. As I said at the beginning of this book, your life is on the precipice of great change. It's up to you!